Pilates

FUSION

well-being for body, mind, and spirit

By *Shirley Sugimura Archer*

Illustrations by Nicole Kaufman

CHRONICLE BOOKS
SAN FRANCISCO

To the spirit of my ancestors from both the East and West.
Thank you for inspiring me to create a bridge that blends the best of
these rich cultures for the benefit of all people.

Library of Congress Cataloging-in-Publication Data available.

ISBN: 0-8118-3987-7

Manufactured in China

Designed by Gayle Chin, Protopod Design

Distributed in Canada by Raincoast Books
9050 Shaughnessy Street
Vancouver, British Columbia V6P 6E5

10 9 8 7 6 5 4 3 2 1

Chronicle Books LLC
85 Second Street
San Francisco, California 94105

www.chroniclebooks.com

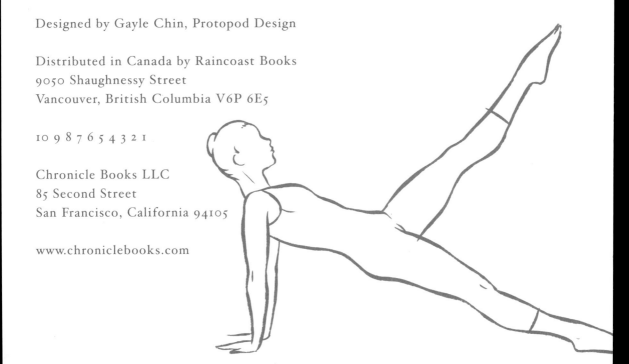

PiLaTeS

FUSION

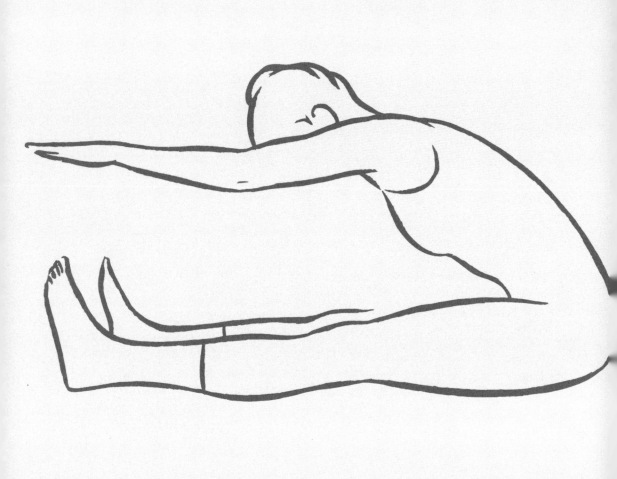

TABLE OF
CoNTeNTS

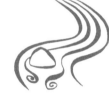

part I

PILATES FuSioN

FOR EVERY BODY

As rivers have their source in some far off fountain,
so the human spirit has its source.
To find this fountain of spirit
is to learn the secret of heaven and earth.

{lao-tsu}

> Physical fitness can neither be acquired by wishful thinking nor by outright purchase.
>
> {Joseph Pilates}

chapter 1

UNDERSTANDING PILATES FuSioN: AN INTRODUCTION

You deserve to get the most out of life. In order to do this, you need to have a healthy body, a clear mind, and a soaring spirit. *Pilates Fusion,* much more than a run-of-the-mill exercise book, aims to teach you what you need to know to condition your body and your mind and to release your inner spirit. By following the simple steps in this book you can be strong, beautiful, fit, and fantastic for life.

It's never too early or too late for you to start feeling your best. Seize the moment and make it yours.

What Is Pilates?

Pilates is a terrific way to get in shape, flatten your stomach, tone up your muscles, and improve your posture. It's also an excellent way to restore your body after pregnancy or improve your sports performance. After practicing a few months, you (and others!) will notice the change in your physique.

The Pilates practice includes exercises performed on a floor mat and exercises done using specialized equipment such as the Reformer, the Trapeze Table, and the Wunda Chair. The Pilates mat practice may be performed alone or be augmented by the use of props or equipment. In an effort to make Pilates accessible to everyone, this book focuses on mat exercises that require a minimal amount of equipment.

The Pilates approach works for everyone because it trains and conditions the deepest muscles at the body's center, or "core." When you train your core muscles, your posture and your body awareness improve. And when you perform the coordinated muscle movement patterns of Pilates, your grace, ease, and efficiency of movement also increase. For most people, this means eliminating back pain and reducing back injuries, not to mention firming up the abdominal and torso muscles. For athletes, it means improving speed and power and reducing injuries.

Pilates targets the core muscles, those internal muscles that we so often forget about when performing conventional workout routines. These muscles stabilize the spine, shoulders, and pelvis. The core muscles lie on top of one another in layers. The deepest muscles stabilize the spinal column and give the brain "position sense" information about where the vertebrae are in space and in relation to the rest of the body. The muscles in the middle layer brace the spinal column, particularly the lower back, helping to prevent injuries. The muscles in the outermost layer move the trunk. When you bend, twist, or rotate, you are using the outer-layer muscles. Exercise and movement professionals refer to these outermost muscles as "global," or "mover," muscles.

Historically, body-building exercises have targeted mover muscles because these muscles lie directly under the skin and are most visible when toned. However, research shows that the most effective core training targets each layer of muscles to optimize spinal stabilization and overall fitness—in effect, "working from the inside out." East Asian movement disciplines such as Tai Chi Chuan (a slow, meditative form of shadow boxing), Qigong, karate, and other martial arts also emphasize training from the body's center, known as *t'an tien* in Chinese and *hara* in Japanese. Joseph Pilates referred to the use of the deeper abdominal muscles as "centering" or strengthening the "powerhouse."

FIND YOUR DEEPER ABDOMINAL MUSCLES

Here's a great exercise to help you distinguish between your deeper stabilizer muscles and your more superficial mover muscles.

1 Stand tall and place your palms on your belly. Inhale and, as you exhale, bend forward slightly. Notice that, as you bent forward using your mover (rectus abdominus) muscles, your belly bulged downward.

2 Stand tall again with your palms on your belly. Inhale and, as you exhale, draw your navel toward your spine, "scooping" your abdominal area. Maintain this muscle action in your abdominals. Inhale again, then exhale and bend forward, keeping your navel lifted up toward your spine. This time notice that, as you bent forward, your belly did not bulge downward but instead stayed up close to your spine.

3 Stand up and relax.

Activating your deeper abdominal muscles kept the belly from bulging. When you perform your Pilates exercises, you will consistently activate the deeper abdominal layer.

Before you begin your Pilates program, assess your posture to create a benchmark against which to measure your progress.

1 Wear minimal, form-fitting clothing so you can see your physique.

2 Stand naturally, facing sideways, in front of a full-length mirror. Turn your head to view yourself in the mirror.

3 Check to see whether your ears and the midpoints of your shoulder, hip, knee, and ankle are in a straight line.

4 Notice whether your lower back is flat, excessively arched, or neutral.

5 Notice whether your palms face the sides of your body or your shoulders round forward with your palms facing back.

After exercising regularly for one month, recheck your posture for any improvement.

When we focus on building only the mover muscles, we create imbalances that can lead to injury and chronic pain. If the inner stabilizer muscles are weak, then the outer mover muscles must assist in stabilization functions. This inefficient, unbalanced division of muscle labor can lead to chronic tension and pain in mover muscles—particularly in the lower-back, neck, and shoulder areas—which are not designed to play a "bracing" role.

An imbalance can also occur when one part of an opposing muscle group (such as the biceps and triceps, or the chest and back muscles) dominates the other due to greater strength. For example, if you sit at a desk all day, your chest and front-shoulder muscles are probably stronger than your upper-back and rear-shoulder muscles, causing your shoulders to round forward.

Pilates exercises can retrain your body's muscles to perform their intended functions; you can condition your stabilizer muscles to stabilize and your mover muscles to move. While the work is subtle and requires attention to detail, you will continue to progress with each exercise session. As your muscles begin to function more efficiently, you'll increase your overall strength and feeling of well-being. Over time, you can transform your entire body.

One visible benefit of Pilates is improved posture, which can make you feel tall and confident and can even make you look thinner. The inner stabilizer muscles targeted in Pilates exercises support the spine and help maintain correct spinal alignment, or "neutral alignment." When the spine is aligned correctly, the ear, shoulder, hip, knee, and ankle line up with each other vertically. The natural, gentle S shape of the spinal column is retained and the discs are not compressed.

When you sit or stand using proper spinal alignment, you avoid back pain and pinching of nerves that run through the spinal column. Improper alignment can lead to chronic mus-

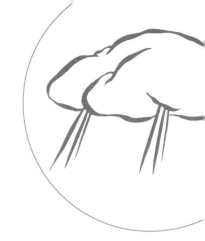

cular tension, headaches, restricted blood flow, pinched nerves, faulty breathing patterns, poor digestion, and reduced overall health and well-being. You can assess your posture with the "Quick Posture Check" on the facing page.

All in all, practicing Pilates will benefit your health, energy, and appearance. Over time, you will notice increased strength in your back, abdominal, and pelvic-floor muscles; as a result your posture will improve, making you look taller and slimmer. The muscles of your legs, hips, shoulders, chest, and arms will become toned, giving you added flexibility and strength. This additional strength will energize you throughout each day and your increased flexibility will give you ease and grace as you move. With continued practice you'll find that your metabolism increases, which in turn will cause your energy to increase, so that you can be more active.

Who Was Joseph Pilates?

The Pilates exercise program was invented by a man who firmly believed that a lack of physical activity undermines physical health. In the "good old days," people needed to exert more energy just to get through the day and keep food on the table. Our lives today are not as physically demanding. Weakness, stiffness, and weight gain result. It's not our fault. Our modern environments simply do not demand that we physically exert ourselves to survive.

Joseph Hubertus Pilates was born in 1880 in Dusseldorf, Germany. During his childhood, he suffered from asthma, rickets, and rheumatic fever. To improve his health, the determined young man turned to physical training. He took up diving, skiing, gymnastics, and bodybuilding. By the time he reached the age of fourteen, his physique was so well developed that he worked as a model for anatomical charts.

Joseph Pilates invented several apparatuses to complement his exercises. Some of his inventions include the following:

Reformer
Inspired by a hospital bed, the Reformer features a sliding carriage that rests on top of a large rectangular frame upon four legs. At one end of the frame is a foot bar. Two straps can be looped around the feet or hands for exercise variations involving arm and leg movements. Springs attached to the carriage and frame provide resistance.

Trapeze Table
(also called Trap Table)
Pilates created the Trapeze Table while being held in a British internment camp, where he attached bedsprings to walls above hospital beds to provide patients with a way to exercise while bedridden. The Trapeze Table resembles a table with four metal posts connected at the top by a rectangular frame. At one end is a spring-loaded "push-through bar." At the other end are a variety of springs and a hanging bar that looks like a trapeze.

continued on page 13

During World War I he worked in a hospital while detained as an enemy alien in British internment camps. There he worked to develop physical conditioning methods to rehabilitate those confined to bed. He created training equipment from beds, using bedsprings to facilitate exercise. These inventions formed the basis for the now-popular Reformer, which still resembles a cot, and for the Trapeze Table, which looks like a table with hanging springs and bars.

After the war, Pilates returned to Germany. There he met Rudolph von Laban, a choreographer, who incorporated some of Pilates' methods into his own teaching. Modern dance pioneer Hanya Holm learned these exercises from von Laban and included them in her dance class warm-ups. In 1926, Pilates immigrated to New York, where he opened a physical fitness studio. Pilates' clientele included George Balanchine, Martha Graham, Ted Shawn, Ruth St. Denis, and Ron Fletcher, among others. Balanchine was a strong advocate of the benefits of Pilates' method and invited Pilates to train dancers in the New York City Ballet. Today, many Pilates exercises remain a staple of dance conditioning.

Over the years, Joseph Pilates' apprentices continued to develop his work and incorporate their own influences. Now, variations of the Pilates method are practiced around the globe and millions of people from all walks of life enjoy the conditioning benefits of this form of exercise. What unites the various strands of the Pilates method is the adherence to the basic principles and a love for the work itself.

What Is Pilates Fusion?

With its focus on flowing movement patterns and breathing techniques, Pilates is similar to ancient Eastern mind-body practices such as Yoga, Tai Chi Chuan, and martial arts. But Pilates is neither a spiritual nor an intuitive practice. Rather, the purpose of Pilates training is to improve the physique.

The Pilates method reflects its modern Western influence in its emphasis on the use of will and the rational mind; Joseph Pilates named his system of exercise Contrology because he believed that conscious control of muscular movements could lead to physical perfection, health, and happiness. However, today, in addition to physical wellness, we need mental wellness to manage stress, relax, and stay centered. That's where *Pilates Fusion* comes in. It melds the best of the Pilates practice with Eastern philosophy.

More and more we hear about the mind-body-spirit connection. But what is it really? Eastern medicine and exercise disciplines use a holistic approach that takes into account the health of the body, mind, and spirit. Traditional Chinese medicine addresses both emotional and physical symptoms. Ancient treatments such as acupuncture restore the flow of healthy life energy and bring the body, mind, and spirit back into a state of balance. The same can be said of Eastern exercise disciplines such as yoga, Tai Chi Chuan, Qigong, and martial arts. These disciplines focus not only on perfecting physical movements but also on restoring balance to the mind, the body, and the spirit.

The Western medical research community has long been investigating the power of the mind-and-body relationship to improve and promote health. Current research in preventive medicine and exercise science corroborates the benefits of Eastern forms of mind-body training. Studies confirm that Tai Chi Chuan and yoga improve physical health, sleep, and stress and anger management; decrease pain and pain sensitivity; and instill a greater sense of well-being.

In the West, the mind-body focus of Eastern disciplines offers a *new* training approach. The Pilates Fusion program presented in this book combines the Western ideals of rational and scientific attention to movement with the Eastern concept of holistic health. By including Eastern-inspired concepts in your approach to exercise, you can experience the immediate

PILATES' REVOLUTIONARY INVENTIONS

Wunda Chair

Pilates intended this exercise tool to double as a household chair when not in use. It resembles a step stool with a padded seat. Attached to the inside of the stool is a bar with springs. To perform exercises on the Wunda Chair one pushes the spring-loaded bar up and down with either the feet or the hands. Poles can be added to the sides to provide arm support for exercises performed when standing on top of the chair.

While these tools are very helpful to stabilize the body while strengthening and lengthening the muscles, you can achieve similar results with the mat exercises.

If you have difficulty seeing images in your mind's eye or you don't enjoy doing visualizations, simply focus on your breath and your physical sensations. The skill of visualizing, like any skill, improves with practice. Be patient and view it as a tool that serves you in a positive way, not as a source of frustration. Find a harmonious balance that's effective for you.

benefits of awakening your spirit as you cultivate the more gradual physical changes that will result from your Pilates practice. In this process you will strengthen not only your body, but also the balance and flow of your own life-force energy.

To help you make the mind-body-spirit connections as you practice, I've included a "Spirit" cue for each exercise. These cues offer inspiring visualization ideas to help you awaken your spirit, develop awareness of your body's vital energy, and see yourself as part of the scheme of all living beings.

Visualization works because the mind processes mental images in the same manner that it processes actual experiences. As you see and experience yourself in your mind's eye, your body will follow. And when you perform each exercise and connect your mind both with your body's energy *and* with the life energy of the natural, living world, you increase your sense of your own place on the planet. You see yourself as a part of the whole universe of life, rather than as an isolated being. This connects you with your deepest level of inner calm and tranquility.

As you continue your practice, you'll find that your awareness of your inner self and your external environment is heightened. Over time, you will start to notice when you hunch your shoulders, grind your teeth, or clench your fists, actions that may have previously gone unobserved. You'll tune in to your natural signals of fatigue, tension, energy, and even hunger. You will be able to detect subtle cues that signal potential injuries before they become more serious problems.

While toning up your body you will unite your physical self with your inner being—you will find greater connectedness between your mind, body, and spirit. In Eastern traditions, masters who are believed to have attained the highest state of mental development are those who can keep their mental focus continuously in the present, which is actually much more difficult than it sounds. Many of us, consciously or unconsciously, spend a great deal of our time worrying about

tomorrow or ruminating about the past. When we are preoccu-
pied with our thoughts, we are not truly experiencing the present
moment. We are living more in our mind than in our body.
We miss out on what is happening here and now. Practicing
Pilates Fusion will help you learn to clear your mind and
focus on the present.

This journey to increased self-awareness is one of the
most rewarding aspects of your practice. When I'm teaching,
I continually remind my students that their most powerful
work is accomplished when they are off the mat and away
from the training room. When you find yourself applying the
lessons of your Pilates exercises while you sit at your desk,
on your couch, or in your car while stuck in traffic, you will
have begun your true transformation. You no longer mindlessly
slouch, putting pressure on your spinal discs and compressing
your internal organs. Instead, you stand or sit up tall and
proud, feeling calm, relaxed, and at ease with yourself.

Your Pilates Fusion program is *not* simply about end
results and achieving goals; it's about enjoying the process.
It's about feeling pleasure and joy in movement as an affirmation of your own life-force energy—and of your place in the
wondrous scheme of all living things. This exercise program is
a potent part of your own self-care. Your health and well-being
lies within you. All you need to do is make a commitment to
draw it out. As you practice, congratulate yourself each day
for taking steps to realize your potential and live more fully.

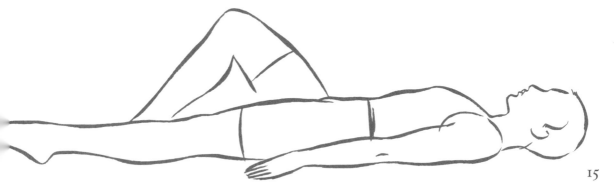

Research has shown that when people concentrate on the muscles they are training they achieve more rapid results. As you prepare for each and every movement during your workout, mentally review not only your technique but also your image of yourself performing the exercise. Visualize the movement, see your strong and healthy muscles, and feel the heat generated by your own power. When you concentrate, your workout will fly by and you will finish with a great sense of accomplishment.

One study found that participants who communicated positive messages to their muscles were able to work harder and achieve more gains. Fill your mind with positive thoughts, reminding yourself of everything that you can achieve. Avoid saying, "I'm so tired. I'm never going to make it." Instead, tell yourself, "I feel my strength. I'm doing great. I'm doing the best I can at this moment."

How to Use This Book

My intention with *Pilates Fusion* is to outline simple steps for those who want to try Pilates but find it hard to fit new activities into their lives. By breaking down the exercises into simple steps and offering visualizations to free the inner spirit, I aim to make Pilates an easy and enriching fitness program for everyone.

Anything we can do to make wellness a priority in our lives will have a positive effect on our health, even if we can spare only a few minutes a day. I've included basic exercises that you can practice if you have just a few minutes, along with more advanced exercises and recommended exercise sequences. *Pilates Fusion* won't restrict you with rules and regulations. Rather, the book will show you how to adapt the practice to your busy lifestyle. So, whether you have ten minutes or a whole hour, you'll get the maximum benefit for your time. And you'll feel good about taking small steps every day, an approach that will have a powerful impact in the long run.

Use the exercises in this book in the manner that best suits you. If you prefer to focus solely on physical training, you will condition your muscles and improve your mind-body connection and body awareness. If you choose to work on a deeper level and explore and strengthen your own inner energy, then you can use the visualization, relaxation, and deep-breathing exercises to connect with your inner spirit.

Now, set aside any worries about your current fitness level and abilities. It doesn't matter whether you are fit or experienced in exercise. What matters is that you simply embrace who you are and begin.

chapter 2

GETTING STaRTeD:
TAKING THE FIRST STEPS

When practiced correctly, Pilates yields many physical and mental benefits. To ensure that you get the maximum benefits and also avoid injury, you'll need to take care of a few details before you begin your exercises. In this section you'll find all the information you'll need to get off to a smooth, comfortable start.

Talk with Your Health-Care Provider

Safety should come first with any exercise program. If you are a man over the age of forty-five or a woman over the age of fifty-five, if you are pregnant, or if you have any other medical condition, you'll need to find out if you have special physical needs before starting any exercise program. Many people with chronic conditions can exercise safely as long as they do so within specific limitations. Consult your health-care provider for advice on your situation.

I'm a firm believer that the benefits of regular exercise far outweigh any risks involved. Experts agree that even for frail older adults, the risks of physical activity are less than the risks of being completely inactive. As long as you respect the limitations of your body, and follow your health-care provider's advice, you will be doing yourself a world of good.

Create a Practice Space

Once you've determined that you can safely begin your exercise program, you'll need to create a practice space. It's no fun to move furniture around or clear the floor before every

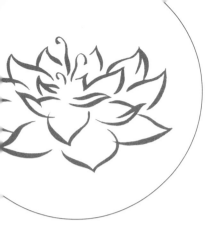

movement session. So try to find a space, even a small one, just for Pilates. When you have a designated practice space it's easier to stick to a regular workout schedule. You'll enjoy returning to your own special, inviting spot time after time, to practice, center yourself, and restore your energy. Respect your space and ask those you live with to also respect it.

In your practice space, you'll need enough room to lie down, lift your legs up and to the sides, and stretch your arms overhead and out to the sides. Remove any furniture that could get in your way; since most of the exercises require dynamic movements, it's all too easy to hit an arm or leg against a nearby table or chair. If you like to check your posture visually, a mirror is useful, but it's not essential.

Keep an eye on climate control. Make sure your practice space is adequately ventilated and neither too warm nor too cold. A room that is too chilly can cause you to tense your muscles and prevent you from reaping the benefits of your workout. As you improve your muscle tone and body awareness, you'll perform more vigorous movements that will elevate your body temperature, so if the climate is warm, you may want to use a fan to keep you cool and circulate the air.

Preparing your practice setting is essential to your peace of mind. When you're ready to do your exercises, prepare yourself both physically and mentally for a focused movement session. Eliminate as many distractions as possible. Don't respond to knocks on the front door. Let the answering machine take phone calls. Close doors to your space to keep pets or children at bay. Put soothing background music on a continuous-play mode to create a peaceful mood. Making these preparations will enhance your concentration and, as a result, prevent injuries caused by sudden movements in response to distractions.

Wear Proper Practice Clothing

When you exercise, it's essential that you feel comfortable and able to move easily. Fabrics that breathe and dry quickly, such as soft cotton or synthetic, are ideal. It's up to you to decide whether to wear loose or clinging clothing. Form-fitting clothes do not impede movement and they allow you to check your alignment in a mirror. Clothing made with Lycra supports your muscles, keeps them warm, and enhances circulation (as long as they are not too tight). Loose clothes allow freedom of movement and feel cool on hot days. Pants with soft, wide waistbands and unitards without a waistband are the most comfortable garments to wear while exercising on your back. Avoid clothing with buttons, snaps, or zippers that could rub or chafe. Generally, wear what makes you feel good.

Since Pilates mat exercises are low impact, athletic bras or jock straps are not essential. Shoes are not necessary. In fact, performing exercises barefoot makes it easier for your feet to connect with the ground and helps to prevent slipping.

Choose the Right Exercise Mat

Thick mats, thin mats, hard mats, soft mats—which mat is right for you? Pilates mat exercises often involve rolling on your back or stomach. These rolling movements are much more comfortable with adequate cushioning, particularly if you do not have a lot of natural padding on your body. On the other hand, a mat that is too soft can make it difficult for you to tell whether you are maintaining neutral spinal alignment when you are lying down. You need some firmness under your body to help you differentiate the curves of your spine from points of contact on the mat.

While performing Pilates mat exercises does not require a lot of equipment, certain props can enhance your progress or comfort.

• **Five-inch Ball**
A small ball may be placed between thighs or ankles to encourage the use of the pelvic-floor and inner-thigh muscles and to actively engage muscles in the midline of the body.

• **Magic Circle**
Designed by Joseph Pilates, the Magic Circle consists of a metal ring with cushioned pads on two opposing sides and is used to create resistance when held between the legs, arms, or hands.

• **Exercise Band**
A wide elasticized band usually four to five feet in length can be used to create resistance when held in the hands and placed around the body.

• **Foam Roller**
A foam roller can be placed under the back when lying down, or under the hands or feet. It's used to challenge core stabilizer muscles to maintain balance and to enhance stretching and strengthening exercises.

• **Stretching Strap**
Such a strap enhances stretching of tight muscles. A fabric strap approximately six feet long and one inch wide works best.

• **Foam Wedge**
This type of wedge alleviates pressure when placed under wrists for exercises such as push-ups. It also assists in maintaining a neutral pelvis position in seated exercises when placed under the pelvis.

Choose a high-quality sticky mat that is at least three-eighths of an inch thick and lay a towel on top of it. A one-eighth-inch-thick sticky mat is generally too thin. firm, dense foam mats may be too hard when used alone, but they may be effective when paired with a sticky mat or a towel.

Your mat is an investment that will significantly affect your comfort and enjoyment of your exercises. Sample different mats at your fitness center or see if the sporting goods store has models you can try. Or, if you work with a trainer, he or she may be able to obtain a high-quality mat for you.

Mat hygiene is also important. Avoid sharing mats with strangers since you can develop skin infections from contacting fungus on a mat, or if bacteria on a mat come into contact with a cut or sore on your skin. Clean your mat regularly with soap and water. Allow your mat to dry before rolling it up. Some mats are even made with antibacterial materials, although these mats are more expensive.

The only other item that is essential for your exercise program is a towel. You can lay a towel on your mat to provide additional cushioning and absorb perspiration. In the Curl-Up with Hammock (page 42), you can use your towel to assist you as you curl up and engage your abdominal muscles. If you have muscular tightness in your neck, upper back, and shoulders or if you have a thick back, you may need to put a rolled or folded towel under your head as a pillow so as to maintain neutral neck alignment. In side-lying positions, you may use a towel as a pillow under your head or to support your waist.

Now you are prepared to begin the exercises. But before you start, I will offer tips on how to move safely in order to avoid injury. Pilates exercises can be modified to accommodate many individual needs. By remembering to work at the appropriate level and taking your time to progress gradually, you will succeed during every exercise session.

Essential Training Principles

Joseph Pilates drew on yoga, boxing, and even Chinese acrobatics, among other movement styles, to develop his exercises. What distinguishes Pilates is its incorporation of the following six principles:

- Control
- Concentration
- The "powerhouse"
- Precision
- Flowing movement
- Breathing

I've incorporated the following four additional concepts into the Pilates Fusion approach:

- Neutral spine
- Life-force energy
- Harmony
- Fusion of body, mind, and spirit

These four concepts add a further dimension to traditional Pilates. Pilates experts disagree on the definition of true Pilates. Some purists believe that the exercises must be presented exactly as Joseph Pilates taught them. Others believe that the exercises may depart somewhat from their original form as long as they remain true to the fundamental principles and spirit of the work. I believe it is a testament to the strength of Joseph Pilates' work that this fitness program can stand the test of time and evolve with modern influences. Let's explore these concepts further.

CONTROL

The principle of control is the foundation upon which Pilates is built. Joseph Pilates believed that a few repetitions of an exercise, executed with control and concentration, provided better training than numerous repetitions done carelessly.

CONCENTRATION

Correct execution of Pilates exercises involves highly specific movement patterns. Some exercises even require you to focus your attention simultaneously on different parts of your body, which can be challenging at first. Contemporary research has found that concentrating on movement is healthy for the brain. Studies suggest that regular physical activity, because it stimulates the brain and the neuromuscular system to perform coordinated patterns, helps to prevent or deter the onset of diseases that impair cognitive faculties in older adults.

THE "POWERHOUSE"

The "powerhouse" is the physical center of the body—the area between the bottom of the rib cage and the hip bones. The muscles in this part of the body support the spine and internal organs and affect posture. Most Pilates exercises require you to stabilize the powerhouse before executing arm, leg, and torso movements.

PRECISION

Precise execution of every aspect of each exercise is vital in Pilates. The principle of precision works in conjunction with the principles of concentration and control. As Joseph Pilates recommended, "Concentrate on the correct movements each time you exercise, lest you do them improperly and thus lose all the vital benefits of their value. Correctly executed and mastered to the point of subconscious reaction, these exercises will bring grace and balance in your routine activities." With precise attention to subtle movements you can train your body and mind to work more efficiently.

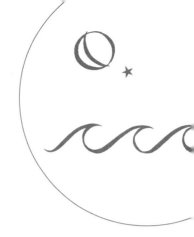

FLOWING MOVEMENT

Pilates is meant to be performed in a fluid, natural manner without "jerky starts and sudden stops." The principle of flowing movement complements the principles of concentration, control, and precision. After you learn to focus your mind on your body, you must then learn to release excess tension, so your movements are smooth and flowing. This aspect of Pilates practice probably stems from traditional East Asian movement disciplines such as Yoga, Tai Chi Chuan, and Qigong, which incorporate the concepts of fluid motion, strength, flexibility, and balance.

BREATHING

Pilates was a strong proponent of breath as a vehicle to energize the body. Each exercise is meant to be performed with full inhalations and exhalations. Pilates advised, "Squeeze out the lungs as you would wring a wet towel dry. Soon the entire body is charged with fresh oxygen from toes to fingertips, just as the head of steam in a boiler rushes to every radiator in the house." Each Pilates exercise coordinates movement patterns with breathing patterns, a fundamental feature of Pilates exercises.

   Joseph Pilates passed away in 1967, but his work has endured, evolved, and remained vital as new generations of teachers have incorporated additional concepts to address contemporary lifestyles. I've added the following four concepts to create the Pilates Fusion approach, which embraces modern living and Eastern philosophies.

NEUTRAL SPINE

Technology has all but removed necessary physical activity from our lives. The result is a collapsed upper body, characterized by rounded shoulders and a short, tight neck. Preserving the natural curves in the spine is essential for optimal health. Moira Stott of Stott Pilates™ in Toronto, Canada, promotes

In traditional Chinese medicine, the Mind and Body include three treasures of Life: Mind, Chi (also called Qi or Ki), and Essence. Chi is considered the natural life force that exists in all life forms and connects them to each other in the natural world.

the concept of supporting and strengthening the natural alignment of the spine, referred to as "neutral spine" or "neutral alignment." The exercises in this book incorporate ways to protect and develop a healthy neutral posture.

LIFE-FORCE ENERGY

The concept of life-force energy, the idea that all living things possess a universal, connecting energy, is rooted in holistic Eastern philosophies, in which humans are seen as a part of this natural living world. As you perform each exercise and follow the accompanying Spirit cue, you can strengthen your awareness of your own inner energy and focus on restoring its healthy balance and flow. You'll become more attuned to the life-force energy pulsing within you and throughout nature and you'll appreciate your mind and body's potential to be strong, limber, alert, and relaxed.

HARMONY

As you increase your body awareness, you will find yourself learning to move more in harmony with your body. As you establish this unity of mind and body, so will you feel more at peace with yourself and with life. With practice, you'll improve your ability to tap into this deep sense of calm regardless of your outside circumstances.

FUSION OF EASTERN PHILOSOPHY AND WESTERN PHYSICAL TRAINING

The cornerstone of this book's approach to Pilates exercise is *fusion*. Fusion is the union of separate things by melting or blending. It is the creation of something new.

Blending, or fusing, the best of Joseph Pilates' exercises with the ideas of Eastern philosophy gives you a powerful new focus for your life—one that will help you to live positively, affirm your well-being, and discover the connectedness of your body, mind, and spirit. Through fusion, you gain the benefits of Western physical training and the wisdom of the Eastern mindset.

Strength of body, clarity of mind, and freedom of your inner spirit are your rewards from your Pilates Fusion practice. Build your body's strength. Increase your body's agility. Cultivate the clarity and flexibility of your mind. In so doing, you will support your long, healthy, and balanced life.

Injury Prevention

You've undoubtedly heard the phrase "no pain, no gain." In fact, most of us have heard it so many times we've come to believe that if an exercise doesn't hurt, then it's not working. Unfortunately, untold numbers of injuries result when people ignore their body's pain signals and overdo their exercise. In the East, attitudes toward exercise for health are vastly different. Traditional Eastern movement practices favor honoring and respecting the body. Taking this gentler approach allows you to accept yourself as you are and act in harmony with nature, which automatically minimizes injuries.

Compared with many sports, Pilates comes with a very low risk of injury. However, Pilates exercises do involve spinal movements, so you must use particular care if you have spinal, joint, or other musculoskeletal conditions. When performed correctly, Pilates exercises strengthen the muscles that support the spine and can alleviate or even prevent back pain. The key is to listen to your body and progress gradually.

The neck is a particularly vulnerable area of the spine. The neck and shoulder stabilizer muscles should support the head, which weighs approximately ten pounds, as a natural extension of the spine. A sedentary lifestyle, however, contributes to a slouched posture and weak neck and shoulder muscles. As a result, we tend to hold our head level as we round the chest forward, leading to shortening of muscles in

As you train, you'll need to understand the difference between "good" pain and "bad" pain. Bad pain is your body's way of letting you know that something is wrong. If you move in a particular way and feel a sharp or severe pain, pay attention: this is your body's signal to stop that movement.

Good pain, in contrast, is not really pain but rather the discomfort associated with fatigue—it's telling your body that your muscles are tired because they have worked hard. Good pain tends to be felt in a generalized area rather than in a specific spot. As you progress with your Pilates exercises, this discomfort will cease to feel like pain. Instead, your muscles will feel awake and alive and glad to be used. You may even start to look forward to this feeling.

the back of the neck. If your neck feels fatigued or strained when you exercise, protect it by supporting your head with your hand or using a towel as a hammock to assist your neck muscles. (See Curl-Up with Hammock exercise, page 42, to learn how to do this.) Practicing exercises such as Curl-Up with Hammock (page 42), Curl-Up with Long Arms (page 43), and the Hundred 1 (page 44) will strengthen your neck over time. See page 50 for additional neck-strengthening suggestions.

The lower back also requires special attention. Eight out of ten adults in the United States experience lower-back pain at some point during their life. Back pain is a leading cause of workplace absenteeism and a source of chronic discomfort for many. Fortunately, regular practice of Pilates strengthens muscles that support the lower back. To avoid injury, maintain a neutral pelvic position as recommended in the exercise instructions, and avoid progressing to more advanced moves until you are certain that you can stabilize your pelvis. Attempting exercises that are too difficult may cause you to arch your back, straining it in the process. If you can progress gradually and take care of your back, you will prevent injury and strengthen key postural muscles. You will also feel taller, leaner, and more powerful.

Since Pilates requires concentration and physical effort, refrain from exercising when you are not feeling well. Don't exercise if you're taking painkillers or any other medications that could impair your judgment. Also, avoid working out for two hours after you eat. A full stomach can make core conditioning (which involves the muscles around the abdomen) quite uncomfortable.

Before exercising, warm up your body, beginning with breathing exercises and progressing from foundation exercises to more rigorous movements. This is particularly important if you are exercising first thing in the morning or after a long day spent sitting at your desk. Muscles, joints, and connective tissue such as tendons and ligaments tend to be stiff and tight in the morning, and stiffness tends to become more pronounced as you age. Sitting at a desk all day tends to tighten the lower back, neck, and shoulders.

Think about the best time of day for you to practice. Morning workouts are a wonderful way to greet the day and increase alertness. Pilates exercises awaken your spine and enhance your attention to your movements throughout the day. Your body changes from day to day, so turning your attention inward as you wake up can give you a sense of what your body needs. Be particularly sensitive to any areas of stiffness and move conservatively, gradually bringing your activity and energy levels up. At the end of your morning session, breathe deeply and draw in energy as you enjoy a total body stretch.

Performing Pilates at the end of the day requires a somewhat different warm-up. While your body may be more flexible in the evening than it is in the morning, your mind may be less peaceful, your attention having been focused on meeting obligations and solving problems all day. When I teach evening classes, I spend more time on breathing exercises and focusing attention inward to increase awareness of physical sensations. Make your evening exercise a time for you to let go of daily stresses and worries, connect with yourself, and restore your energy. Pay particular attention to warming up and stretching the lower back, since it can become tight and compressed from sitting for long periods of time. Closing an evening session with a thorough body stretch and relaxing meditation is a wonderful way to bring your energy down and prepare for a restful evening.

WHAT CAUSES BACK PAIN?

The majority of back pain results from trauma to the spine from compression, tension, or shearing forces. Common movements, such as lifting a heavy weight or pulling on something from an awkward position, can lead to painful muscle strains and spasms. The part of the spine located in the lower back is most vulnerable when twisting and bending motions are combined. These sorts of movements, done incorrectly, can cause trauma to the vertebrae, discs, or ligaments. Practicing your Pilates foundation exercises will retrain your body to move more efficiently. Over time, you will strengthen your deep postural muscles, helping you to avoid back injury.

Remember to honor, appreciate, and accept your body just as it is. Many of us look in the mirror and feel only frustration and disappointment. Our society puts a high value on physical perfection, so it's no wonder we feel discouraged when our bodies don't match up to that ideal. But keep in mind that healthy bodies come in all shapes and sizes. What's important is not a supermodel-perfect thigh (which may be digitally enhanced in photographs anyway) but the strength and flexibility of that thigh. Through Pilates or any other exercise program you won't achieve a picture-perfect body, but you can work to make your body strong, lithe, and healthy.

Honoring your body means learning the basic exercises before progressing to a higher level of difficulty. Respect each exercise for what you can learn and gain from it. Taking one level at a time, gradually training the correct muscles, will eventually enable you to perform the most advanced exercises. This process requires mental discipline, but the benefits are worth the effort. The wonderful thing about the human body is that if you practice consistently, you will become stronger. So, take your time, respect your body, and have faith in the process.

Your body is a marvelous miracle. It allows you to do the work you were meant to do, care for those you love, and feel great sensual pleasure. Quite simply, it is what makes your life possible. Honoring your body means appreciating all that it has done for you and treasuring it as the temple of your spirit. Love and accept it. Be patient with it. Only when you feel self-acceptance can you make true gains in strength—not only physical strength but also inner strength from your own sense of purpose and value.

Everything
is beautiful,
in its own
way.

{Anonymous}

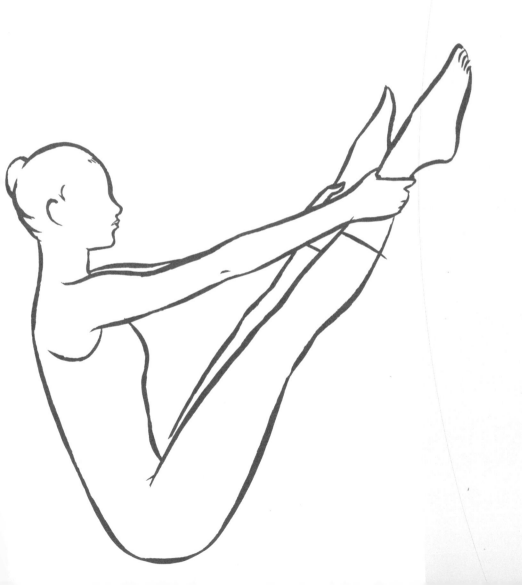

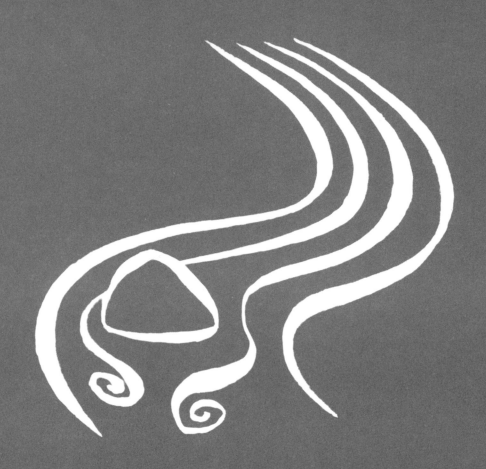

part II

YOUR PiLaTeS

FUSION PROGRAM

Before the first step is taken, the goal is reached.
Before the tongue is moved, the speech is finished.
More than brilliant intuition is needed
to find the origin of the right road.

{Ekai Mumon}

chapter 3

FOUNDATION eXeRCiSeS:
LAYING THE GROUNDWOR

> ## The mind leads the body.
>
> {Koichi Tohei}

Like erecting a building, developing a strong and stable center begins with the foundation. The Foundation Exercises that follow help you to develop your awareness of the core stabilizer muscles that support good posture and learn how to move your arms and legs while maintaining that posture. They also provide the basis for more advanced Pilates work, such as the Progressive Exercises introduced in chapters 4 and 5. Beginners may use the set of Foundation Exercises as a complete workout or as a training program before moving on to the Progressive Exercises. More experienced fitness enthusiasts can use them to warm up for more difficult moves. Almost everyone can benefit from practicing these basic movement patterns. The particular benefits of each exercise are set forth with the exercise instructions.

Perform five to ten repetitions of each exercise unless indicated otherwise, depending on your strength and energy level. Quality of form is essential, particularly because you are reinforcing new movement habits. During your workout, do not continue an exercise if you cannot maintain correct form. Simply stop, rest, and proceed to the next exercise.

Begin your Pilates journey with the Base Position and the fifteen exercises that follow it.

Base Position

1 Lie on your back, knees bent approximately ninety degrees, feet flat on the ground, heels aligned with sitz (sitting) bones, and arms at your sides with palms down (see Note).

2 Tilt pelvis back until your lower back contacts the ground.

3 Tilt pelvis forward until your back is slightly arched.

4 Lie comfortably between these two extremes in a "neutral pelvis" position.

5 Repeat 5 to 10 times. During the exercise, make sure the entire back of your rib cage maintains contact with the ground. Do not let your lower rib cage arch upward.

6 Slide your shoulders up toward your ears, then down as far as you can. Keep them in the relaxed lower position. Widen shoulder blades and soften your chest and shoulders. Lengthen the back of your neck so your head is not tilted back; chin should be slightly tucked. Put a rolled towel or pillow under your head if you have a thick back or if you experience tightness in your chest and shoulders that causes your neck to arch. Now you have a neutral spinal alignment.

S P i R i T
~ one with nature

As you breathe, feel stability and comfort, strength and peace. Imagine you are practicing amid the beauty of nature. Feel the firmness of the earth beneath you. Enjoy the openness of the sky above you. Soften and open your chest as you become ready to receive today's experience. As body, mind, and spirit become one, so you become one with the natural world that creates all life.

NOTE

Arms are lifted in figures to show spinal alignment. To perform the exercise, place arms at your sides with palms down.

BENEFITS

- Reinforces neutral spinal alignment (result of contact with ground)
- Improves posture
- Improves spinal stability

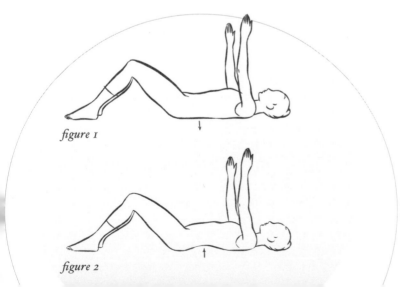

figure 1

figure 2

Bring your awareness to the present. Notice the rhythmic flow of your breath. Feel your body move as it breathes. Pilates breathing raises energy in your body's center. With each inhalation, feel your breath energizing you. With each exhalation, feel strength and power in your body's center increase as you release what you no longer need.

LISTEN TO YOUR BODY

Avoid overbreathing. If you are new to breathing exercises, you may "overbreathe" and feel dizzy as a result of hyperventilation. Stop doing breathing exercises if you start to feel light-headed. Breathe naturally instead. As you become accustomed to breathing deeply, overbreathing should not be a problem. If you take medications to reduce hypertension or if you have diabetes, breathing exercises may not be appropriate for you. Talk with your health-care provider.

Pilates Breathing

1 Lie on your back in Base Position (page 33) with knees bent ninety degrees, feet flat on the ground, and arms with palms placed on sides and top of your lower rib cage.

2 Inhale and exhale naturally, observing any movements of your torso.

3 Inhale, feeling your ribs as they expand wide and connect with the ground.

4 Exhale, pulling your pelvic floor upward as you contract your rib cage.

5 Next, inhale and exhale slowly and deeply, using your deep abdominal muscles, contracting your lower rib cage inward and pulling your navel toward your spine.

6 Continue breathing. With each inhalation, gently allow air to flow in and feel your rib cage expand. Contract your pelvic floor and deep abdominal muscles as you exhale and feel your rib cage contract.

7 Repeat 5 breath cycles. (One inhalation and one exhalation equals one breath cycle.)

Variation
• Sit comfortably in your chair and place your hands on the sides of your lower rib cage with your thumbs on your back and your fingers on the front of your body. Inhale and exhale as described above and notice the expansion and narrowing of your ribs with your breath. Repeat 5 times.

- Enhances mind-body connection

- Conditions deep abdominal muscles

- Improves flexibility of rib cage

- Strengthens respiratory muscles

- Increases energy

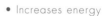

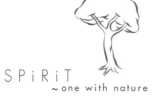

Imagine that your breath is an energizing wind bathing every cell in your body. As you exhale, your breath carries away what you no longer need. Feel the natural lengthening of your spine as you inhale. Feel the spine contract as you exhale. Allow your pelvis to arc naturally as your breath ebbs and flows.

NOTE

Arms are lifted in figures to show spinal alignment. To perform the exercise, place arms at your sides with palms down.

LISTEN TO YOUR BODY

Stop if you feel any pain or discomfort. Relax your shoulders and soften your chest. Try to move easily and without tension. Practice focusing your mind without tensing your body.

BENEFITS

- Releases lower-back tension
- Increases awareness of subtle spinal movements occurring with the breath
- Conditions deep abdominal muscles

Pelvic Tilt

1 Lie on your back in Base Position (page 33) with knees bent ninety degrees, feet flat on the ground, and arms at your sides with palms down (see Note).

2 Inhale; remain in neutral pelvis position, between a flat-back and an arched-back position.

3 Exhale as you pull your navel toward your spine. Feel your pelvis tilt back toward the ground. The hip bones and rib cage move toward each other, shortening the waist and "imprinting" the spine on the ground.

4 Inhale as you return to neutral pelvis position and lengthen your waist.

5 Repeat 5 to 10 times.

Note

This movement is subtle. If you're having a hard time identifying it, exaggerate it. Inhale; feel the tip of your tailbone against the ground. Exhale as you flatten back down. When you have identified the arcing pelvis motion, make it smaller. Try to use your abdominal muscles and not the strong muscles of your buttocks to draw your lower back toward the ground.

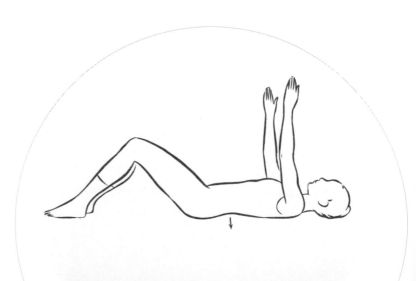

Pelvic Clock

1 Lie on your back in Base Position (page 33) with knees bent ninety degrees, feet flat on the ground, and arms at your sides with palms down.

2 Imagine a clock face on your lower back: twelve o'clock is behind your navel; three o'clock is behind your left hip; six o'clock is the tip of your tailbone; nine o'clock is behind your right hip.

3 Inhale as you roll your pelvis up onto six o'clock. Exhale as you press the clock points of your lower back in a clockwise motion against the ground. Keep feet, knees, and legs as still as possible. Feel your abdominal muscles working.

4 Perform 4 or 5 clockwise circles, then reverse direction.

SPiRiT
~ one with nature

Sense the awakening of the power in your body's center. Imagine a soft, glowing light just beneath your navel growing larger and brighter with each repetition. Feel heat begin to rise in your powerhouse, or center, as your muscles become energized.

LISTEN TO YOUR BODY

Stop if you feel any pain or discomfort. Relax your shoulders and soften your chest. Avoid clenching your jaw, tightening your throat, or curling your toes. Concentrate on practicing your movements without tensing your body.

BENEFITS

- Enhances the mind-body connection
- Improves lower-back mobility
- Conditions abdominal muscles, especially the oblique muscles
- Massages lower-back
- Releases lower-back tension

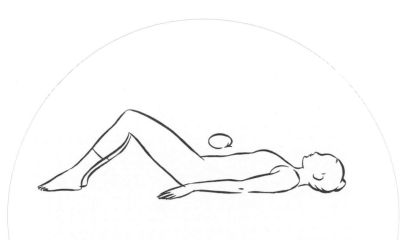

Connect the soles of your feet with the earth beneath you. As you peel your spine off the ground, feel energy flowing through your body as you open your chest and back wide and lift your powerhouse, or center, up toward the sky and lower it back down to the ground. Sense the merging of your energy with the life energy surrounding you.

LISTEN TO YOUR BODY

Stop if you have any lower-back pain or discomfort. Return to Pelvic Tilt (page 36) until you grow stronger. Perform Knee Hug Stretch (page 96) to release any tension from your lower back.

BENEFITS

- Improves spinal mobility, especially in the lower back

- Strengthens muscles in the abdomen, hamstrings, and buttocks

- Tones hips and back of thighs

- Conditions pelvic stabilizers

- Stretches the lower back, releasing tension

Bridge

1 Lie on your back in Base Position (page 33) with knees bent ninety degrees, feet flat on the ground, and arms at your sides with palms down.

2 Move heels closer to hips and slide your shoulders down. Exhale as you begin slowly to tilt up your pelvis, lifting your lower back off the ground.

3 Continue peeling your spine off the ground, one vertebra at a time, stopping when you reach your shoulders. Inhale and hold neutral spinal alignment; allow your weight to rest on your shoulders and feet.

4 Exhale as you slowly roll down, one vertebra at a time, to Base Position (page 33).

Variation
• **Add Rib Cage Arms (page 40) movements while you are in the elevated bridge position. Return arms to your sides before lowering your body back to Base Position (page 33).**

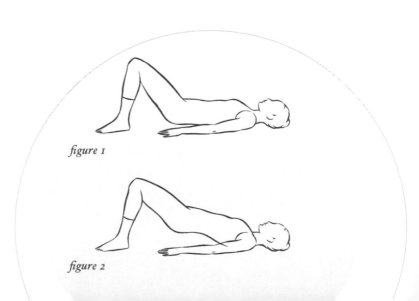

figure 1

figure 2

Shoulder Slaps

1 Lie on your back in Base Position (page 33) with knees bent ninety degrees, feet flat on the ground, and arms at your sides with palms down.

2 Inhale as you lift both arms straight up above your shoulders, rotating palms inward.

3 Exhale and relax, feeling the contact of your shoulder blades with the ground.

4 Breathing naturally, reach one arm and then the other up toward the sky by lifting and dropping one shoulder blade and then the other, gently "slapping" the shoulder blades against the ground.

5 Feel a stretch between the shoulder blades in the upper middle back. Feel your scapula move and slide across your back as you lift your arms one at a time.

6 Repeat 5 to 10 times.

7 To finish, soften and relax your chest, then inhale. As you exhale, bring your arms down to rest at your sides in Base Position (page 33).

SPiRiT
~ one with nature

Imagine a soft, glowing light in your upper body. Feel this light expand and grow brighter, as energy streams out through your fingertips to touch the sky. Experience the pull of gravity as your shoulder slaps back onto the ground.

BENEFITS

- Opens up back and chest
- Improves shoulder mobility
- Enhances awareness of shoulder placement and scapular stabilization

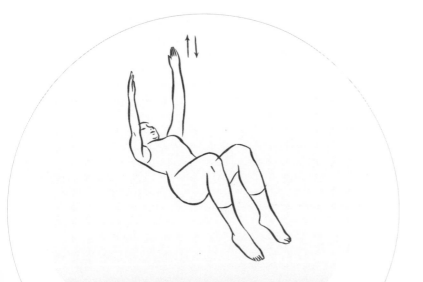

Imagine you can touch the sky with your fingertips. As you reach up toward the heavens, feel the support of the earth beneath you, keeping you grounded. Feel your connection with the openness of the sky and the stability of the ground.

LISTEN TO YOUR BODY

Keep your movements within a range that is comfortable for you. Don't arch your back or your neck. Stop if you feel any neck or shoulder pain or discomfort.

BENEFITS

- Opens up chest and straightens rounded shoulders
- Improves shoulder stabilization
- Conditions deep abdominal muscles
- Improves posture

Rib Cage Arms

1 Lie on your back in Base Position (page 33) with knees bent ninety degrees, feet flat on the ground, and arms at your sides with palms down.

2 Inhale as you lift both arms straight up above your shoulders, rotating palms inward.

3 Exhale as you continue the arcing motion overhead, extending your arms past your ears in a gentle V shape. Do not hunch your shoulders. Keep the rib cage grounded—only extend your arms as far as you can without lifting your ribs off the ground. Feel your stabilizer muscles working to maintain a neutral spine. Feel a stretch in your chest and in the front of your shoulders.

4 Inhale as you arc arms upward again, palms facing inward. Keep your rib cage against the ground.

5 Exhale as you continue to arc your arms back down to your sides, palms down, returning to Base Position (page 33).

6 Repeat 5 to 10 times.

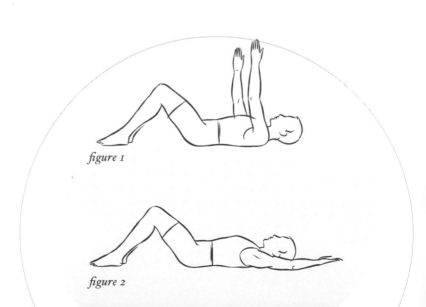

figure 1

figure 2

Leg Slides

1 Lie on your back in Base Position (page 33) with knees bent ninety degrees, feet flat on the ground, and arms at your sides with palms down.

2 Inhale. Exhale as you extend one leg by sliding the heel away from pelvis. Only slide the heel as far as possible without moving the pelvis. Avoid both arching and flattening your back. Feel your stabilizer muscles working to maintain a neutral spine.

3 Inhale. Exhale as you pull your heel back to Base Position (page 33) without moving pelvis.

4 Repeat with the other leg.

5 Alternating legs, repeat 5 to 10 times.

Variation
• **Inhale. Exhale as you slide your heel out; inhale as you pull your heel in.**

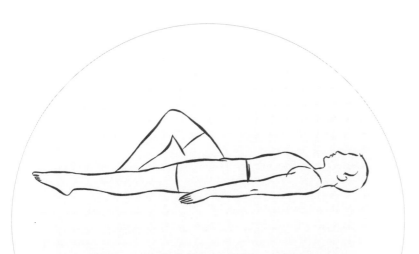

SPiRiT
~ one with nature

Feel the stability and strength of the solid earth beneath you. As you move your leg, draw the earth energy up into your body's center of power. With each repetition, bathe your core in earth energy, feeling strong, centered, and stable.

LISTEN TO YOUR BODY

Avoid excessive tension. Focus your energy on targeted muscles. Do not clench your jaw or throat or hunch your shoulders. Soften your chest. If you feel a lot of tension in the upper thighs, stop and stretch your body with the Full-Length Torso Stretch (page 98).

BENEFITS

• Improves pelvic stabilization

• Conditions deep abdominal and spinal stabilizers and pelvic-floor muscles

• Improves posture

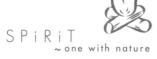

Feel energy rise in your
body's powerhouse, or center,
just below your navel.
Imagine a warm, glowing
light in your center that grows
stronger and brighter with
each repetition. Feel your
own strength and power rise
with the brilliance of the
glowing light.

LISTEN TO YOUR BODY

Do not pull on your neck or
hunch your shoulders. Perform
the Knee Hug Stretch (page
96) to release any tension
from your lower back. Do the
Full-Length Torso Stretch (page
98) to stretch your abdominal
muscles afterward, if necessary.

BENEFITS

- Increases awareness of
  neck and shoulder tension

- Lengthens neck

- Encourages shoulder
  relaxation

- Strengthens abdominal
  muscles

Curl-Up with Hammock

1 Place a towel or mat on the floor. Lie on your back in Base Position (page 33) with knees bent ninety degrees, feet flat on the ground, and arms at your sides with palms down. The towel or mat should be underneath your middle back, extending beyond the top of your head. This is your hammock.

2 Reach overhead and take an edge of the towel with each hand.

3 Inhale. Exhale as you curl up your upper body, allowing the weight of your head to rest on the towel hammock. Feel your abdominal muscles contract, particularly below the breastbone.

4 Inhale as you roll down.

5 Repeat 5 to 10 times.

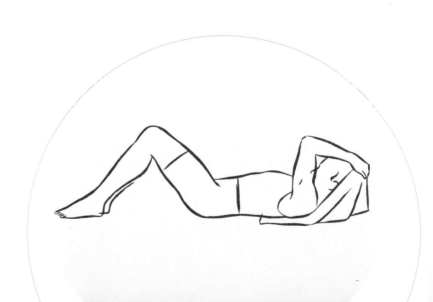

Curl-Up with Long Arms

1 Lie on your back in Base Position (page 33) with knees bent ninety degrees, feet flat on the ground, and arms at your sides with palms down.

2 Exhale as you slide your shoulder blades down to stabilize your shoulders and open your chest. Keep your shoulders relaxed.

3 Exhale as you curl up your upper body, fingertips reaching toward ankles. Feel your abdominal muscles contract, particularly below the breastbone.

4 Inhale as you roll down.

5 Repeat 5 to 10 times.

SPiRiT
~ one with nature

Imagine increasing your power with each repetition. Feel the heat grow in your body's powerhouse, or center, just below your navel. Imagine a shining sun in your center that grows more brilliant as your strength increases.

LISTEN TO YOUR BODY

If you feel any neck pain or discomfort, support your head with one hand, with your elbow pointing outward and your upper arm as flat as possible to keep the chest open. Switch the supporting hand if necessary for comfort. Perform the Knee Hug Stretch (page 96) to release any tension from your lower back. Do the Full-Length Torso Stretch (page 98) to stretch your abdominals afterward, if necessary.

BENEFITS

- Opens up chest and back and straightens rounded shoulders
- Conditions shoulder stabilizers and neck muscles
- Strengthens abdominal muscles

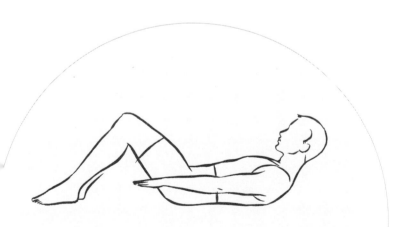

Imagine burning embers in your body's powerhouse, or center, growing brighter with each breath cycle. Feel your inner strength and power expanding within the fire's glow.

LISTEN TO YOUR BODY

If you feel any neck pain or discomfort, support your head with one hand, with your elbow pointing outward and your upper arm as flat as possible to keep the chest open. Perform arm beats with your other arm. Switch arms after five breath cycles.

BENEFITS

- Strengthens and tones abdominal muscles

- Conditions pelvic and shoulder stabilizers and neck muscles

- Reinforces neutral spinal alignment

- Raises energy level and invigorates

* NOTE

This movement prepares you for The Hundred II (page 53).

The Hundred I*

1 Lie on your back in Base Position (page 33) with knees bent ninety degrees, feet flat on the ground, and arms at your sides with palms down.

2 Exhale as you slide your shoulder blades down to stabilize your shoulders and open your chest.

3 Exhale as you curl up your upper body, fingertips reaching toward ankles. Feel your abdominal muscles contract, particularly below the breastbone. Hold the position for the entire exercise.

4 Pump arms up and down, about two to three inches, 5 times as you inhale. Then pump arms up and down, about two to three inches, 5 times as you exhale. Each breath cycle (one inhalation and exhalation) features 10 arm pumps, or beats.

5 Repeat for 10 breath cycles, if you can. (The 10 arm beats multiplied by 10 breath cycles equal 100 arm beats, which is how this exercise gets its name.)

Variation
• To remind yourself to keep your chest and back open, keep your palms up as you inhale, and keep palms down as you exhale.

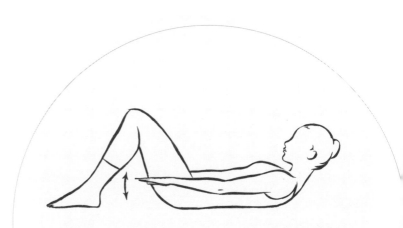

Plank *

1 Lie face down, legs straight. Place your elbows under your shoulders; rest your forearms on the ground with palms facing inward and hands in gentle fists. Slide your shoulder blades down to stabilize your shoulders. Lengthen the back of your neck.

2 Pull in your abdominal muscles to stabilize torso and lift rib cage. Do not arch your back. Make sure your body weight is distributed between your elbows, forearms, hips, and tops of legs. Work up to a 30-second hold.

Variation
• To increase difficulty, continue to lift up onto your knees, maintaining the length in your spine. Make sure your body weight is distributed between your elbows and forearms and knees. Work up to a 30-second hold.

• To further increase difficulty, curl your toes under and push up onto the toes and balls of feet. Distribute your body weight evenly among points of contact with the ground. Avoid putting most of your body weight on your elbows. Work up to a 30-second hold.

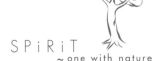

SPiRiT
~ one with nature

Imagine that you have a central beam as strong as a thick tree trunk running through the center of your body. Picture your muscles wrapping around this beam like vines wrapping around the trunk of a tree; continue to breathe and embrace that strong and solid center.

LISTEN TO YOUR BODY

If you feel any shoulder pain or discomfort, perform only the easiest version. Do the Shell Stretch (page 99) and Cat Stretch (page 100) to stretch the abdominal and back muscles afterward.

BENEFITS

• Conditions shoulder, spinal, and pelvic stabilizer muscles

• Reinforces neutral spinal alignment

• Improves posture

• Improves self-confidence

* NOTE

This movement prepares you for the Leg Pull, Facing Down (page 79).

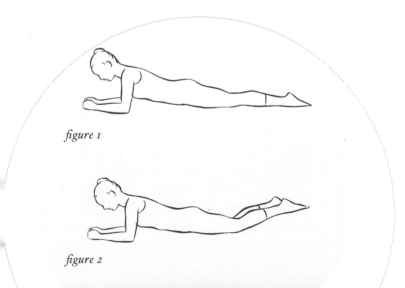

figure 1

figure 2

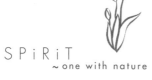

SPiRiT
~ one with nature

Inhale and draw in energy. Exhale and power yourself up, drawing on the earth's energy to strengthen your will and power of concentration.

LISTEN TO YOUR BODY

If you feel any wrist pain or discomfort, place a rolled towel under your palms, allowing your fingers to touch the ground. Elevating your palms relieves wrist pressure. If your knees are uncomfortable, place a towel under them for additional cushioning.

BENEFITS

- Strengthens chest, shoulders, and arms
- Conditions abdominal, spinal, and pelvic stabilizer muscles
- Reinforces neutral spinal alignment
- Improves posture

Modified Push-Up

1 Kneel on all fours with hands under your shoulders and knees under hips, in a "table" position. Place your hands slightly wider than chest-width apart. Slide your shoulder blades down to stabilize your shoulders. Lengthen the back of your neck. Pull abdominal muscles in to stabilize the torso and lift the rib cage. Do not arch your back or hunch your shoulders.

2 Walk your knees away from your torso and lengthen your spine and upper thighs like an inclined plank. Keep your neck long. Do not lift your hips higher than your shoulders.

3 Inhale as you bend your elbows and lower your chest toward the ground.

4 Exhale as you push your body back up to return to the inclined-plank position.

5 Repeat 5 to 12 times.

Variation
• **If you need help keeping your shoulders down and back or keeping your torso long like a plank, make the exercise easier by performing it from the start position.**

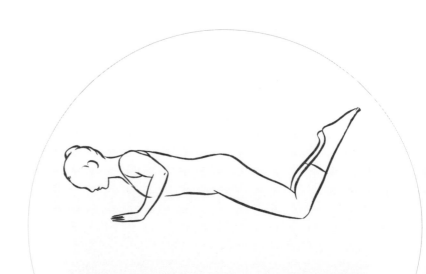

Shoulder Bridge Prep *

1 Lie on your back with a neutral spine, with knees up, feet on the ground in line with hips, and heels as close to hips as is comfortable. The shoulders are relaxed, and arms are at your sides with palms down.

2 Make sure your feet are firmly on the ground. Exhale as you push through your feet and lift your hips up, squeezing your buttocks and hamstring muscles. Allow your weight to rest on your shoulders and feet in the Bridge position (page 38).

3 Inhale as you lower your hips to about one inch above the ground, keeping neutral spinal alignment. Do not shorten your waist or arch your back.

4 Repeat 5 to 12 times.

Variations
• To increase difficulty, in the Bridge position lift one leg up with the knee bent ninety degrees so that the upper thigh is perpendicular to the ground and the shin is parallel to the ground. Perform repetitions keeping only one foot on the ground. Repeat with the other foot.

• To further increase difficulty, fully extend the lifted leg.

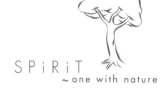

SPiRiT
~ one with nature

Draw the energy of the earth up through your feet as you push off the ground and lift your body's powerhouse, or center, upward, connecting with the energy of the sky and opening your heart center. Imagine that your spine is a tall, strong tree trunk, keeping you solid and centered.

LISTEN TO YOUR BODY

If you feel any back pain or discomfort, do not perform this exercise until you become stronger. Do the Bridge (page 38) to build strength. Perform the Knee Hug Stretch (page 96) to release any tension from your lower back.

BENEFITS

• Strengthens buttocks and hamstring muscles

• Conditions spinal and pelvic stabilizer muscles and abdominal muscles

• Reinforces neutral spinal alignment

• Tones hips and back of thighs

* NOTE

This movement strengthens your buttocks and hamstrings and prepares you for the Shoulder Bridge (page 86).

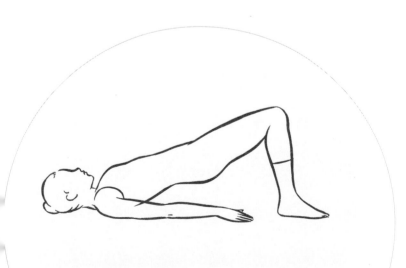

As you arc your top arm above you, imagine that you are painting a rainbow across the sky. Open your chest and back wide as you let energy from the earth and sky stream through your body. Feel strong, centered, and balanced.

LISTEN TO YOUR BODY

Stop if you feel any shoulder pain or discomfort. Continue practicing the Plank (page 45) and Modified Push-Up (page 46) to build strength.

BENEFITS

- Opens up chest and back
- Strengthens oblique and back muscles
- Conditions spinal and pelvic stabilizer muscles and abdominal muscles
- Tones sides of torso and waist
- Improves self-confidence

*NOTE

This movement prepares you for Side Series: Side Bend (page 72).

Side Bend Prep *

1 Recline on your side, with bottom elbow under your shoulder, and forearm and palm down. The bottom knee is bent ninety degrees, the top leg is straight, and the top arm is in front of body, palm up.

2 Plant your bottom elbow firmly beneath you. Exhale as you push your lower hip up off the ground, keeping the bottom shoulder stabilized and sweeping the top arm in an arc over your head. Do not hunch your shoulders; keep your back and neck long. Pull in your abdominal muscles and keep your buttocks tight to stabilize your pelvis. Keep your chest and back wide.

3 Inhale as you lower your body back to the start position. Keep your torso perpendicular to the ground. Do not rock forward or back.

4 Repeat 5 to 10 times.

5 Repeat on other side.

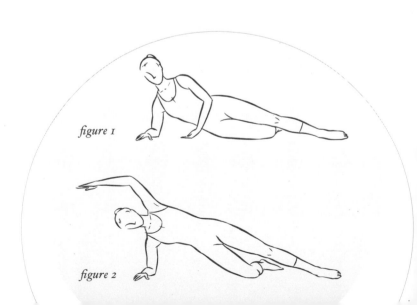

figure 1

figure 2

Leg Pull, Facing Up Prep *

1 Sit with knees bent ninety degrees, feet flat on the ground. Place hands with palms down behind and outside of hips, fingers facing whatever direction is most comfortable.

2 Exhale, pushing your feet firmly into the ground as you lift your torso upward to a "table" position. Squeeze your buttocks and hamstrings to lift your hips. Be sure your feet are under your knees and hands under your shoulders. Straighten your arms without locking your elbows. Stabilize your shoulders. Lift your head to gaze down the front of your torso. Breathe normally.

3 Work up to a 30-second hold.

SPiRiT
~ one with nature

As you push your hands and feet into the ground, imagine the energy of the sun drawing your body's center upward like a plant growing toward the light. Picture your muscles wrapping firmly around your spine like climbing vines, making it stronger. Enjoy the challenge of finding your inner power.

LISTEN TO YOUR BODY

If you feel any wrist pain or discomfort, place a rolled towel under your palms, allowing your fingers to touch the ground. Elevating your palms relieves wrist pressure. Alternatively, try using fists instead of open hands.

BENEFITS

- Opens up chest and straightens rounded shoulders
- Strengthens arm, shoulder, and buttocks muscles
- Conditions spinal and pelvic stabilizer muscles and abdominal muscles

*NOTE

This movement will prepare you for Leg Pull, Facing Up (page 80).

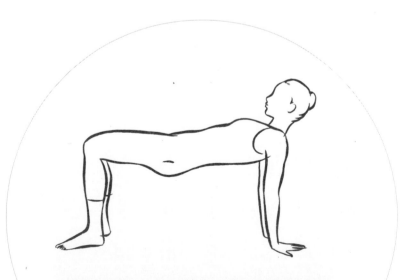

NECK STRENGTHENING EXERCISE

Isometric Neck Press

This exercise strengthens muscles around the neck. It can also help release feelings of tension.

1 Seated in a neutral position, place the palms of both hands behind your head.

2 Inhale. As you exhale, push the back of your head into your hands with backward resistance as you press your hands forward for an isometric contraction. Hold for 6 to 8 seconds.

3 Repeat 5 to 10 times.

Variations:

• Place your palms on your forehead instead of behind your head. Perform as directed, but with forward resistance.

• Place one palm on the side of your head. Perform as directed, but with sideways resistance.

Celebrate Your Wellness

Your Pilates Fusion practice may be benefiting you more than you realize. Be mindful of the positive changes you are making in your life. Take time each day to celebrate your wellness by asking yourself the following questions.

BODY

• Am I feeling stronger?

• Am I feeling more energetic?

• Am I more limber?

• Is my posture improved?

• Do I feel a greater ease of movement?

MIND

• Am I feeling more relaxed?

• Is my concentration improved?

• Am I noticing my posture more?

• Do I have increased awareness of tension in my body?

SPIRIT

- Am I feeling a greater sense of well-being?

- Am I more attuned to my inner voice?

- Do I feel more joy and satisfaction in my life?

- Is there more harmony in my actions, values,
   priorities, and goals?

- Do I have a greater sense of inner peace and serenity?

Neck Glide

This exercise strengthens neck muscles and restores proper alignment of the head and neck. Ideally, you will do this exercise lying down. However, if you're short on time, try it in the car while you're waiting at a stoplight, or try it at your desk when you have a free moment.

1 Inhale. As you exhale, gently flatten the curve in the back of your neck by drawing the chin inward.* Inhale as you return to start position. Imagine that you are growing taller by creating length in the back of your neck.

2 Repeat 5 or 6 times.

* Note: This movement is not a chin tuck, but rather a backward movement of the head so ears are in alignment with the middle of the shoulder.

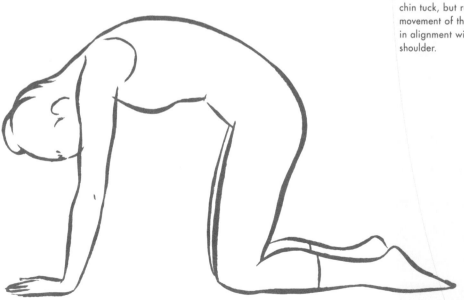

chapter 4
PROGRESSIVE MAT EXERCISES: BUILDING STReNGTH

Once you have mastered the Foundation Exercises and understand how to use your postural stabilizer muscles, you are ready to progress to more difficult movements. The Progressive Mat Exercises will challenge these muscles to improve your strength, flexibility, and coordination. As you continue to practice the Spirit cues, you will enhance your body, mind, and spirit connection.

As with the Foundation Exercises, perform 5 to 10 repetitions of each Progressive Mat Exercise unless indicated otherwise. Focus on quality of movement and on your breathing. Be consistent and patient—you are improving with every workout session.

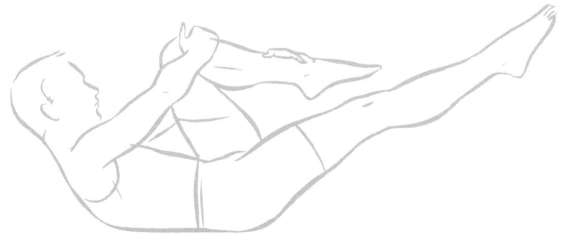

The Hundred II

1 Lie on your back in Base Position (page 33) with knees bent ninety degrees, feet flat on the ground, and arms at your sides with palms down. Lift knees up above hips. Extend one leg, then the other.

2 Inhale as you slide your shoulder blades down to stabilize your shoulders and open your chest.

3 Exhale as you curl up your upper body, reaching arms forward at shoulder height. Feel your abdominal muscles contract, particularly below the breastbone. Hold the position for the entire exercise.

4 Pump arms up and down about two to three inches 5 times as you inhale. Pump arms up and down about two to three inches 5 times as you exhale. Each breath cycle (one inhalation and one exhalation) features 10 arm pumps, or beats.

5 Repeat for 10 breath cycles. (The 10 arm beats multiplied by 10 breath cycles equal 100 arm beats, which is how this exercise gets its name.)

Variation
• To remind yourself to keep your chest and back open, keep your palms up as you inhale, and keep palms down as you exhale.

SPiRiT
~ one with nature

Feel heat increasing in your body's powerhouse, or center, below your navel. Imagine a ball of fire growing larger and brighter with each breath cycle. Feel your inner strength and power within the blaze.

LISTEN TO YOUR BODY

If you feel any neck pain or discomfort, support your head with one hand, with your elbow pointing outward and your upper arm as flat as possible to keep the chest open. Perform arm beats with your other arm. Switch arms after five breath cycles.

BENEFITS

• Strengthens and tones abdominal muscles

• Conditions shoulder and pelvic stabilizer muscles and neck muscles

• Invigorates and raises energy level

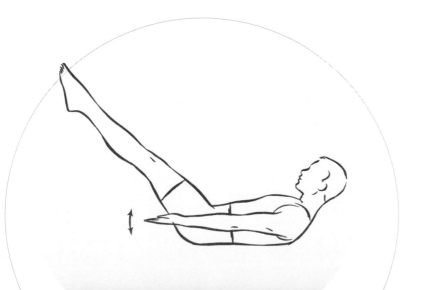

Feel the rhythm in your body that reflects the rhythm of life itself—your breath, your heartbeat, your movements. Imagine that you are an ocean wave flowing up onto shore and back out to sea. Move smoothly, fluidly, and continuously in the steady flow of life.

LISTEN TO YOUR BODY

Stop if you feel any back pain or discomfort. If your lower back is very tight and you cannot sit upright in a neutral position, continue stretching to increase your flexibility. Try the Knee Hug Stretch (page 96), Shell Stretch (page 99), Cat Stretch (page 100), and Deep Buttocks Stretch (page 101) to stretch your back.

BENEFITS

- Strengthens and tones abdominal muscles
- Conditions shoulder stabilizer muscles and neck muscles
- Improves spinal mobility
- Stretches hamstring and back muscles
- Massages the back

Roll-Up

1 Lie on your back in Base Position (page 33) with knees bent ninety degrees, feet flat on the ground, and arms at your sides with palms down.

2 Inhale as you lift both arms upward in an arc without elevating your shoulders. Exhale as you continue moving your arms in the arc, lowering them past your ears. Keep your rib cage grounded.

3 Inhale as you lift both arms back up to the sky. Continue moving, exhale, and keep arcing arms forward as you peel your spine off the ground one vertebra at a time. Pull in your abdominal muscles, flex your feet, and continue to reach forward until your arms are parallel to the floor and your pelvis is in a neutral position. Your neck is lengthened; your gaze is at the ground.

4 Inhale as you lift your upper body. Continue moving, exhaling as you roll your spine down, one vertebra at a time, with your arms naturally falling by your sides and your knees returning to bent position.

5 Repeat 5 to 10 times.

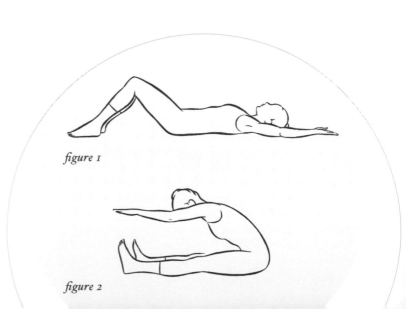

figure 1

figure 2

Leg Circles

1 Lie on your back in Base Position (page 33) with knees bent ninety degrees, feet flat on the ground, and arms at your sides with palms down. Extend one leg straight up. Gently point toes. Relax your shoulders.

2 Stabilize your pelvis in a neutral position. Keep your upper body still and shoulders relaxed. As you complete one breath cycle, move your extended leg clockwise in 5 complete circles, starting with a small circle and gradually increasing its size until it is as large as you can manage while keeping your pelvis stable. Allow your leg bone to glide easily in the hip joint. Do not arch your back or neck or hunch your shoulders.

3 Make 5 circles in the opposite direction.

4 Repeat with the other leg.

Variations

• If you're finding it difficult to keep your pelvis stable, bend the knee of your working leg ninety degrees and make circular movements with your knee instead of your foot.

• If the fronts of your thighs are flexible and you can maintain a neutral pelvis with your leg extended, fully lengthen the nonmoving leg on the ground and use your leg muscles to firmly anchor it in place.

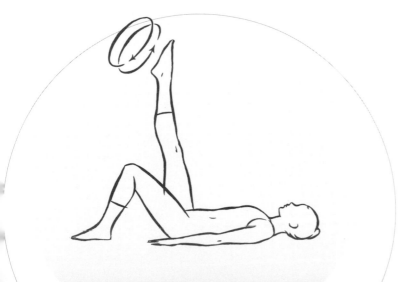

SPiRiT
~ one with nature

Imagine that your hip joint is at the center of a gentle whirlpool. Your leg makes large, smooth circles as it flows with the current. There are no bumps, no edges to the movement—only fluid, consistent motion.

LISTEN TO YOUR BODY

If the backs of your legs are tight, slightly bend the knee of your working leg. To see if your pelvis is moving, place your thumb on your hipbone and your pinkie finger on the ground as you perform this exercise. (You may feel a clicking sound in your joint caused by moving ligaments. As long as it is not painful, it is not harmful.)

BENEFITS

• Improves hip mobility
• Conditions abdominal muscles and pelvic stabilizer muscles
• Strengthens hip flexors
• Tones thighs
• Stretches hamstrings and deep buttocks muscles

LISTEN TO YOUR BODY

Do not roll onto your neck or head. Stop if you cannot control your momentum. If your lower back is tight or rigid, you may be unable to tuck your pelvis under sufficiently to roll. If so, skip this exercise until you become more flexible. Try the Knee Hug Stretch (page 96), Shell Stretch (page 99), Cat Stretch (page 100), and Deep Buttocks Stretch (page 101) to stretch your back.

BENEFITS

- Increases body awareness
- Conditions deep abdominal muscles and shoulder stabilizers
- Stretches the back, especially the lower back
- Massages the back
- Enhances the mind-body connection

Rolling Back

1 Sit on sitz (sitting) bones. Pull both knees toward your chest, gently point feet and place toes on the ground for balance, and place one hand midway down each shin.

2 Inhale as you slide your shoulders down. Exhale as you pull in your abdominal muscles, round your spine, and tilt your pelvis back so you are sitting just behind the sitz bones. Gaze down at your feet.

3 Inhale as you roll onto your shoulders, lifting the sitz bones upward while maintaining the rounded spine.

4 Exhale as you roll back up to the start position, using your deep abdominal muscles to stop before your toes touch the ground.

5 Repeat 6 times.

Variation
• If you are having trouble controlling your momentum, place your hands palms down on the floor beside your hips. Use your hands to assist you by pressing down as you roll back and up.

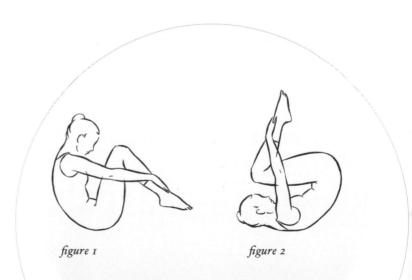

figure 1   *figure 2*

Crisscross

1 Lie on your back in Base Position (page 33) with knees bent ninety degrees, feet flat on the ground; fingertips are held behind head, elbows are out wide, and shoulders are relaxed.

2 Exhale as you lift one, then the other knee above hip joints at ninety degrees. Inhale. Exhale as you rotate upper body to the left lifting your right shoulder toward your left knee, as you draw your left knee in and extend your right leg at a forty-five-degree angle.

3 Pull in your abdominal muscles to stabilize your pelvis. Avoid pulling your neck. Inhale and exhale as you switch legs, rotating each shoulder toward the opposite knee and maintaining the lift in upper body. Inhale as you switch twice; then exhale as you switch twice.

4 Repeat for 5 to 10 breath cycles (one inhalation and one exhalation equal one breath cycle), moving smoothly and rhythmically.

5 To finish, hug both knees to your chest and lower your upper body.

Variation
• If you cannot keep your pelvis still, place both feet on the ground with knees bent ninety degrees. Exhale as you rotate one shoulder toward the opposite knee. Inhale as you roll down through center. Continue, alternating sides, for 5 to 10 repetitions.

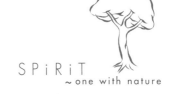

SPiRiT
~ one with nature

Imagine your body's center as the strong trunk of a tree and your chest and shoulders as branches reaching in opposite directions. Feel the length and breadth of your body expand along the trunk and branches.

LISTEN TO YOUR BODY

If you feel any neck or shoulder pain or discomfort, keep your upper body on the ground or skip this exercise. Try the Circle Shoulder, Chest, and Back Stretch (page 102) to improve spinal flexibility.

BENEFITS

• Strengthens abdominal muscles, especially the obliques

• Conditions shoulder and pelvic stabilizers

• Tones abdominal area and waist muscles

• Encourages lengthening of leg muscles

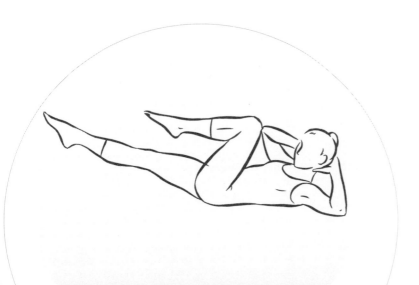

Imagine a beam of light down your body's center extending out to opposite horizons. Lengthen your body along this beam from the top of your head through the tips of your toes. When you are switching legs, slide the insides of your ankles and knees along this beam, lengthening your body and focusing your mind with each repetition.

LISTEN TO YOUR BODY

If you feel any neck or shoulder pain or discomfort, keep your upper body on the ground. Try keeping your head elevated during a couple of switches, then rest your head on the ground for the remainder.

Single Leg Stretch

1 Lie on your back in Base Position (page 33) with knees bent ninety degrees, feet flat, and arms at your sides with palms down.

2 Exhale as you lift the right, then the left knee above hip joints at ninety degrees.

3 Exhale as you pull your navel toward your spine. Feel your pelvis tilt back toward the ground. The hip bones and rib cage move toward each other, shortening your waist and "imprinting" your spine on the ground.

4 Inhale. Exhale as you peel your head and shoulders off the ground, reaching your arms to the outside of your legs.

5 Hold your body in an elevated position. Inhale. Exhale as you extend your left leg at a forty-five-degree angle and draw your right knee toward chest while placing your right hand on your ankle and your left hand on the inside of your right knee. Keep your elbows lifted and wide.

6 Inhale as you switch legs and hand positions twice, pulling the knee toward your chest while extending the other leg. Keep your upper body lifted and pelvis stabilized. Keep your abdominal muscles pulled in. Then exhale as you switch legs twice.

7 Repeat for 5 to 10 breath cycles (one inhalation and one exhalation equal one breath cycle), moving smoothly and rhythmically.

- Strengthens and tones abdominal muscles
- Conditions shoulder and pelvic stabilizer muscles and neck muscles
- Stretches buttocks
- Improves coordination and body awareness
- Encourages lengthening of torso and leg muscles

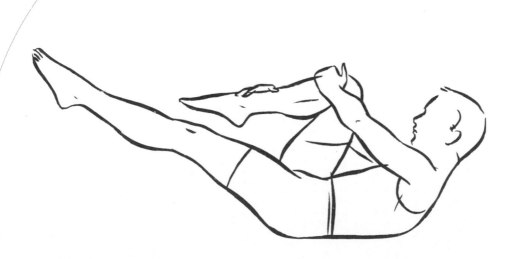

As you extend your arms outward, imagine that you are drawing in life-force energy to rejuvenate your body. Feel this energy surging through your body as you open your heart center to receive all the possibilities of life.

LISTEN TO YOUR BODY

Avoid arching your lower back. If you feel neck or shoulder pain or discomfort, keep your upper body on the ground. Do the Full-Length Torso Stretch (page 98) to stretch your abdominal muscles afterward.

Double Leg Stretch I

1 Lie on your back in Base Position (page 33) with knees bent ninety degrees, feet on the ground, and arms at your sides with palms down.

2 Inhale. Scoop your abdominal muscles toward your spine, exhale as you reach your hands toward your ankles, peel your head and shoulders off the ground, and gaze above your pubic bone.

3 Inhale. Exhale as you lengthen your arms overhead, moving them in an arc to reach past your ears, holding your upper body in an elevated position.

4 Inhale as you circle your arms out and around to the start position at the sides of your legs. Keep your upper body still during arm movements. Keep your shoulders relaxed and abdominal muscles lifted. Only reach your arms overhead as far as you can while maintaining upper-body lift.

5 Repeat 5 to 10 times.

Variations
• For an easier version, keep one knee bent ninety degrees with foot flat on the ground. Halfway through repetitions, switch grounded leg.

• Alternatively, perform exercise with head and shoulders and one leg on the ground.

• See Double Leg Stretch II (page 78).

BENEFITS

- Strengthens and tones abdominal muscles and thighs
- Conditions shoulder and pelvic stabilizer muscles and neck muscles
- Improves shoulder mobility
- Stretches buttocks
- Improves coordination and body awareness

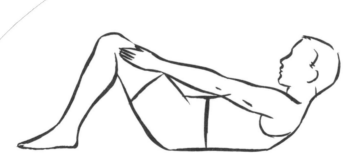

figure 1

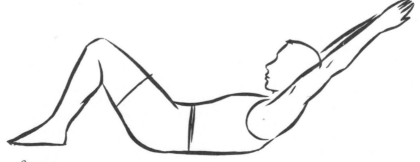

figure 2

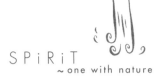

As you bend forward, imagine that you are flowing forward and down from the top of your head like a waterfall. Yield to gravity, relaxing and releasing any tension into the ground, as if water is washing away all of your stress. Then unfurl your spine as you sit upright and imagine that you are blossoming as you are drawn up toward the sun, feeling lighter from having released your tension.

LISTEN TO YOUR BODY

After doing the exercise, shake out your legs and massage the tops of your thighs near your pelvis to relieve any muscle tension.

Spine Stretch

1 Sit with neutral spinal alignment, with straight legs, slightly more than hip-width apart. Rest your hands between your legs, flex your feet, pull in your abdominal muscles, and relax your shoulders. If your pelvis tilts backward, wedge a rolled towel under it to tilt it forward into a neutral position.

2 Exhale as you dive forward headfirst, rounding your spine. Keep your abdominal muscles pulled in to keep sitting bones in contact with the ground and to keep pelvis in a vertical, neutral position. Slide hands forward as flexibility permits.

3 Inhale as you hold the position, relaxing spinal muscles into a stretch and keeping your abdominal muscles tight.

4 Exhale as you round back up, stacking your vertebrae like building blocks, one at a time from the bottom up. Finish in a tall, neutral posture.

5 Repeat 3 to 5 times, moving smoothly and rhythmically.

Variations
• If the backs of your legs are tight, bend knees slightly.

• Sit comfortably in your chair on your sitz (sitting) bones with neutral spinal alignment, with your feet on the ground and shoulders relaxed. Let your arms hang at your sides. As you round forward, allow your arms to fall toward the ground. Perform the exercise. Finish in a tall, neutral posture.

BENEFITS

- Improves spinal mobility
- Conditions pelvic stabilizer muscles
- Tones abdominal muscles
- Stretches neck, back, and hamstring muscles
- Increases body awareness and releases muscular tension
- Enhances the mind-body connection

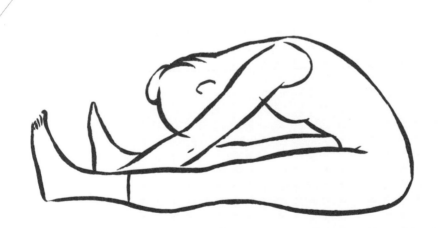

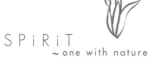

Root your pelvis firmly in the earth. Imagine a central line of energy from the base of your spine to the top of your head. See this energy as a spiraling wind that uplifts your spirit with each rotation, creating feelings of lightness and freedom as you yield and flow, releasing stiffness and rigidity.

LISTEN TO YOUR BODY

After doing the exercise, shake out your legs and massage the tops of your thighs near your pelvis to relieve any muscle tension.

Spine Twist

1 Sit with neutral spinal alignment, legs straight. Flex your feet, pull in your abdominal muscles, relax your shoulders, and place your hands next to your hips. If your pelvis tilts backward, wedge a rolled towel under it to tilt it forward into a neutral position.

2 Exhale as you reach your arms out wide in opposite directions, keeping your shoulders relaxed. Inhale as you lengthen your spine from the top of your head, lifting your ribs away from your hips and lengthening your waist. Feel a sense of openness and lightness between each vertebra in the spine.

3 Exhale as you rotate at the waist for two to three beats, moving slightly farther with each beat. Keep your feet still and your pelvis grounded and facing forward. Do not swing your arms; move from the waist only.

4 Inhale as you revolve, returning smoothly to center.

5 Repeat in the opposite direction.

6 Repeat 3 to 5 times.

Variations

• If you prefer, inhale as you rotate and exhale as you return to center.

• If the backs of your legs are tight, bend your knees slightly.

• If you cannot anchor your straight arms in relation to your shoulders, bend your elbows and touch the pads of your thumbs and fingers together, forming a tentlike shape with your hands. Touch the tips of your thumbs to your breastbone with your elbows out to the sides, relaxing your shoulders.

• Perform the exercise sitting comfortably on your sitz (sitting) bones at the edge of your chair, with neutral spinal alignment, feet on the ground, and shoulders relaxed. Perform exercise.

BENEFITS

- Improves spinal mobility
- Stretches middle and lower back
- Conditions shoulder and pelvic stabilizer muscles
- Tones arms and shoulders

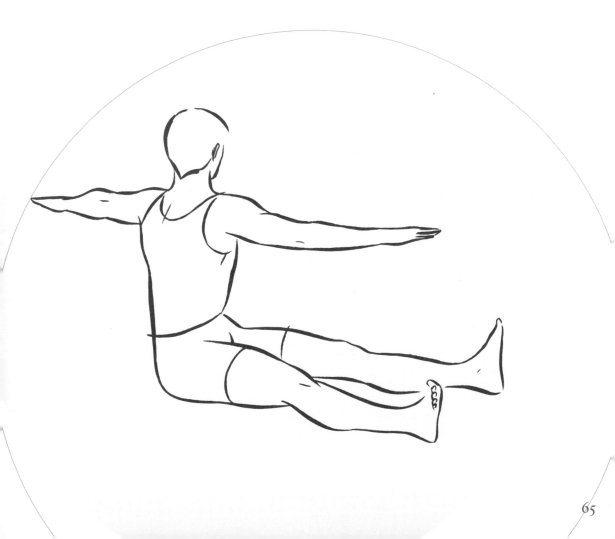

SPiRiT
~ one with nature

Feel the inviting expansiveness of the sky and the firm stability of the earth as you keep your body light and your chest and back open. Breathe in to connect with your body's powerhouse, or center. Exhale and release any limitations on your ability to hold your position and use your inner strength.

LISTEN TO YOUR BODY

Stop if you feel any shoulder or lower-back pain or discomfort.

Side Series: Side Kick

1 Lie on your side; establish a neutral spine position with your pelvis perpendicular to the ground. Pull in your abdominal muscles and lift up your waist so it is not touching the ground. If you let your abdominal muscles relax, your waist will sink into the ground. Rest your head on your outstretched bottom arm, keeping your neck long. Place your top arm on the side of your ribs, bend your elbow ninety degrees, and place your hand on the ground in front of your navel like a kickstand. Keeping your top leg straight without locking your knee, lift the leg to hip level.

2 Inhale as you flex the foot of your top leg. In a smooth and controlled fashion slowly swing the top leg forward as far as possible, keeping your torso still, and pulse your leg twice at end of the range of motion. Do not rock your body forward or backward or lose your neutral spine position.

3 Exhale as you point the foot of your top leg and sweep your leg backward as far as possible without moving your torso, keeping the pelvis in a neutral position.

4 To finish, return your top leg to hip level directly above your lower leg.

5 Repeat 5 to 10 times.

Variations
• To increase difficulty, place your top arm on top of your thigh, keeping your balance as you do the exercise.

• To further challenge your upper-body muscles, place your bottom elbow directly under your shoulder, with your forearm and palm down on the ground. Align your shoulder, hips, and legs in one long downward-slanting line. Bend your bottom knee and rest it on the ground. Keep your top leg straight. Push down into the ground through your elbow as you use your core muscles to lift and hold your hips and upper torso off the ground, balancing on your elbow and knee. Keep your shoulder joint open—avoid collapsing your shoulder onto your arm bone. Perform the exercise as described above.

Note
When performing part or all of the Side Series, perform exercises on pages 66 through 73 first on one side, and then on the other side.

BENEFITS

- Conditions shoulder, spinal, and pelvic stabilizer muscles

- Tones abdominal, hip, and thigh muscles

- Stretches hamstring and hip flexor muscles

- Improves balance, coordination, and concentration

- Integrates core and lower body

- Enhances the mind-body connection and movement control

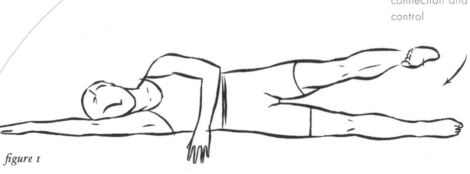

figure 1

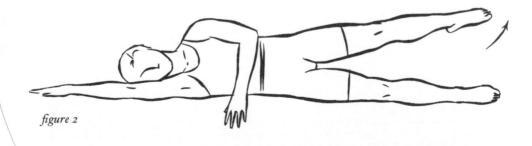

figure 2

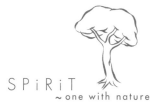

As you inhale, draw in the life-force energy that empowers and strengthens you. Breathe smoothly and evenly, allowing your leg to flow up and down smoothly, appearing effortless like a tree branch swaying in the wind.

LISTEN TO YOUR BODY

If your neck is uncomfortable, place a rolled towel under your head on top of your arm. If you have difficulty maintaining a neutral pelvis and lifting your waist, place a rolled towel under your waist.

Side Series: Outer Thighs

1 Lie on your side; establish a neutral spine position with your pelvis perpendicular to the ground. Pull in your abdominal muscles and lift up your waist so it is not touching the ground. Rest your head on your outstretched bottom arm, keeping your neck long. Place your top arm on the side of your ribs, bend your elbow ninety degrees, and place your hand on the ground in front of your navel like a kickstand. Lift your straight top leg up to hip level.

2 Flex your top foot. Exhale as you lengthen and lift your leg up as high as possible without moving the pelvis. Keep your waist long; pull in your abdominal muscles.

3 Inhale as you lower your leg to join your bottom leg. Maintain a neutral spine throughout the movement.

4 Repeat 5 to 10 times.

Variations
• To increase difficulty, place your top arm on top of your thigh, keeping your balance as you do the exercise.

• To further challenge your upper-body muscles, place your bottom elbow directly under your shoulder, with your forearm and palm down on the ground. Align your shoulder, hips, and legs in one long downward-slanting line. Bend your bottom knee and rest it on the ground. Keep your top leg straight. Push down into the ground through your elbow as you use your core muscles to lift and hold your hips and upper torso off the ground, balancing on your elbow and knee. Keep your shoulder joint open—avoid collapsing your shoulder onto your arm bone. Perform the exercise as described.

Note
When performing part or all of the Side Series, perform exercises on pages 66 through 73 first on one side, and then on the other side.

BENEFITS

- Strengthens outer thighs
- Conditions shoulder, spinal, and pelvic stabilizer muscles
- Tones abdominal, hip, and thigh muscles
- Encourages lengthening of legs
- Integrates core and lower body

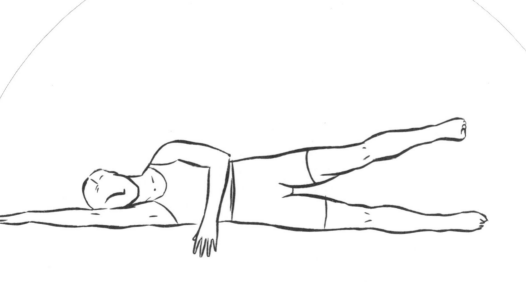

Concentrate on stabilizing your powerhouse, or center, as you lengthen and use the strength in your legs. Notice your ability to experience your entire body at once, truly cultivating your body-mind connection.

LISTEN TO YOUR BODY

If your neck is uncomfortable, place a rolled towel under your head on top of your arm. If you have difficulty maintaining a neutral pelvis and lifting your waist, place a rolled towel under your waist.

BENEFITS

- Strengthens inner thighs
- Conditions shoulder, spinal, and pelvic stabilizer muscles
- Tones abdominal, hip, and thigh muscles
- Encourages lengthening of legs
- Integrates core and lower body

Side Series: Inner Thighs

1 Lie on your side; establish a neutral spine position with your pelvis perpendicular to the ground. Pull in your abdominal muscles and lift up your waist so it is not touching the ground. Rest your head on your outstretched bottom arm, keeping your neck long. Place your top arm on the side of your ribs, bend your elbow ninety degrees, and place your hand on the ground in front of your navel like a kickstand. Lift your top leg slightly wider than your hip.

2 Gently point your toes and rotate both legs so heels are inward and kneecaps face outward. Exhale as you lengthen and lift the heel of your bottom leg to meet the heel of your top leg. Keep your waist long; pull in your abdominal muscles.

3 Inhale as you lower your leg. Maintain a neutral spine throughout the movement.

4 Repeat 5 to 10 times.

Variation
• For an easier version, instead of lifting your top leg to hip level, place the foot of your top leg either in front of your lower leg or behind it, with your top knee bent. Perform the exercise as described.

Note
When performing part or all of the Side Series, perform exercises on pages 66 through 73 first on one side, and then on the other side.

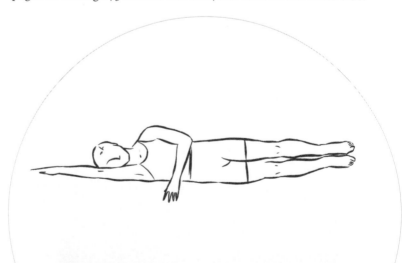

Side Series: Waist

1 Lie on your side; establish a neutral spine position with your pelvis perpendicular to the ground. Pull in your abdominal muscles and lift up your waist so it is not touching the ground. Rest your head on your outstretched bottom arm, keeping your neck long. Place your top arm with palm down on your top leg.

2 Gently point toes, keeping heels together. Exhale as you lengthen and simultaneously lift both legs and upper body off the ground in a "smile" shape. Slide your top hand down your thigh toward your feet, drawing ribs toward hips. Avoid falling backward or forward.

3 Inhale as you lower your legs and upper body back to a neutral spine position.

4 Repeat 5 to 10 times.

Variations
• For an easier version, keep your upper body on the ground. Lift and lower your legs only.

• For an even easier version, place top arm on the ground in front of your body like a kickstand. Lift and lower your legs only.

Note
When performing part or all of the Side Series, perform exercises on pages 66 through 73 first on one side, and then on the other side.

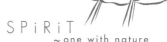
Imagine a line of energy streaming through the middle of your body. As you bend and contract your waist, imagine that you are effortlessly floating up into a warm, beaming smile. Send this warm smile to every cell in your body as you appreciate your body's strength and grace.

LISTEN TO YOUR BODY

If your neck is uncomfortable, place a rolled towel under your head on top of your arm.

BENEFITS

• Strengthens waist

• Conditions shoulder, spinal, and pelvic stabilizer muscles

• Tones hip, thigh, and abdominal muscles, especially the waist

• Enhances the mind-body and upper- and lower-body connections

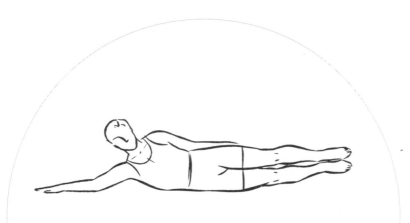

Press your hand firmly beneath you, drawing strength up into your body. As you arc your arm above, imagine that you are painting rainbows across the sky. Open your chest and back wide as you feel the energy of the earth and sky stream through your body.

LISTEN TO YOUR BODY

Stop if you feel shoulder pain or discomfort. To improve wrist comfort, instead of placing your palm flat on the ground, place a rolled towel or a thin mat under your palm, with fingers touching the ground, to reduce severity of wrist angle.

Side Series: Side Bend

1 Recline on your side, with a straight arm and your palm on the ground directly under your shoulder and with your chest open wide. The bottom knee is bent up to ninety degrees as needed for additional support (the more the knee is bent, the easier the exercise becomes, as less balance is required), the top leg is straight, and the top arm is in front of body, palm up.

2 Exhale and push your palm into the ground, lifting your hips up into a neutral spine position, leaving both feet on the ground as you sweep your top arm in an arc up and over your head. Balance your weight through your palm and the sides of your feet. Do not hunch your shoulders; keep your back and neck long. Pull in your abdominal muscles and keep your buttocks tight to stabilize your pelvis. Do not collapse your shoulder. Keep your chest and back wide.

3 Inhale as you lower your body to the start position. Keep your chest facing directly forward. Do not rock forward or back.

Variations
• **For an easier version, lift up onto bottom knee, instead of the side of the bottom foot.**

• **To increase difficulty, in the start position, begin with both legs straight and your top foot in front of the bottom foot. As you exhale and push into the ground, lift your hips and knees, balancing your body on your feet and palm.**

Note
When performing part or all of the Side Series, perform exercises on pages 66 through 73 first on one side, and then on the other side.

- Strengthens waist, shoulders, hips, and thighs
- Conditions shoulder, spinal, and pelvic stabilizer muscles
- Stretches back and sides of torso
- Improves posture
- Enhances the mind-body connection and integrates the entire body

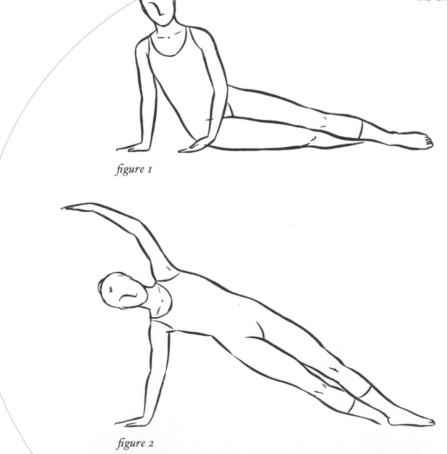

figure 1

figure 2

First, connect your pelvis with the earth. Then imagine that you are a bird soaring upward as you are lifted by the wind. With each lift, allow your chest and back to float skyward, lengthening and lifting like a bird in flight.

LISTEN TO YOUR BODY

Stop if you experience back pain or discomfort or are unable to stabilize your pelvis. To stretch the abdominal and back muscles after this exercise, do the Shell Stretch (page 99) and Cat Stretch (page 100).

BENEFITS

- Opens up chest and straightens rounded shoulders

- Strengthens and tones back muscles

- Conditions back, neck, shoulder, and pelvic stabilizer muscles

- Increases spinal mobility

- Improves posture

Chest Raise

1   Lie facedown, with arms out and palms down. Bend elbows ninety degrees, so that your arms, together with your head, form an E shape. Rotate feet inward. Pull in your abdominal muscles to support a neutral pelvis position.

2   Exhale as you lift upper body and arms without moving pelvis, lengthening spine upward.

3   Inhale as you lower to the start position.

4   Repeat 5 to 10 times.

Variation
• **For an easier version, keep your arms on the ground. Do not push your hands down as you lift; simply rest your arms as if they were floating on the surface of water.**

• **To increase difficulty, extend arms out in a Y shape, with palms facing inward. Avoid hunching shoulders. Slide shoulder blades down and use shoulder stabilizer muscles to keep shoulders in place. Perform the exercise as described.**

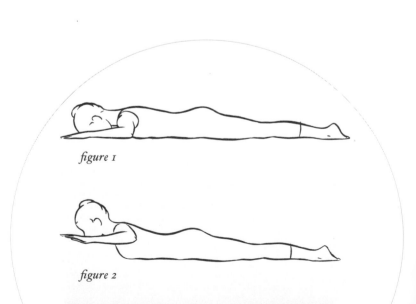

figure 1

figure 2

Leg Lifts

1 Lie facedown, resting head on hands, with legs extended and kneecaps touching the ground.

2 Gently point toes. Exhale as you pull in your abdominal muscles to establish a neutral pelvis position.

3 Inhale. Exhale, keeping your pelvis stable and squeezing your buttocks, as you lift one leg off the ground. Be careful not to arch your back or bend your knees.

4 Inhale as you lower the leg.

5 Repeat with that leg 5 to 10 times and then switch legs, or alternate each leg for 5 to 10 repetitions.

Variations
• To check whether you are maintaining a neutral pelvis position, take the hand on the same side of your body as the working leg and place it palm up on the small of your back. Pay particular attention to your lower back. Do not arch your back or hike your hip up toward the ribs. If feel your lower back or hips moving, you lose your neutral position and you are no longer training your pelvic stabilizer muscles.

• When your abdominal muscles and pelvic-floor muscles are strong enough to stabilize your pelvis, lift both legs off the ground. Do not progress to this level until you can lift one leg 10 times without arching your back.

SPiRiT
~ one with nature

Connect with your body's powerhouse, or center. Imagine a line of energy streaming from your center out through the soles of your feet. With each lift, imagine streaming energy all the way out to the distant horizon, lengthening and strengthening your legs.

LISTEN TO YOUR BODY
Stop if you feel lower-back pain or discomfort. Practice Shoulder Bridge Prep (page 47) to build strength.

BENEFITS
• Strengthens buttocks and hamstring muscles

• Tones buttocks, hips, and thighs

• Conditions spinal and pelvic stabilizer muscles

• Enhances mind-body connection and integrates core with lower body

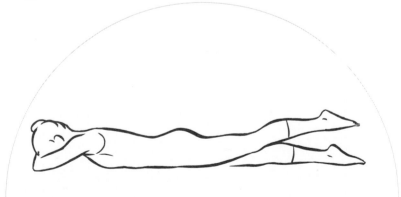

> The journey of ten thousand miles begins with a single step.
>
> {Traditional Chinese Saying}

PuSHiNG YOUR LIMITS

When you have mastered the beginning and progressive exercises and find yourself craving more challenge, introduce the following exercises into your routines. Some of these exercises increase the level of resistance and therefore result in additional strength gains. Other exercises challenge the same muscles but from slightly different angles and in different movement patterns, resulting in improved coordination and a better mind-body connection. You can also use these more advanced exercises to cultivate your awareness of life energy in your body.

Continue to challenge your mind and body and deepen your understanding of life-force energy with the following ten exercises.

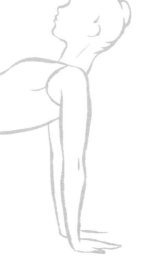

Modified Swan Dive

1 Lie facedown, legs straight. Roll heels in and knees out, gently point your toes, and place your hands beside your shoulders, palms down.

2 Inhale as you slide your shoulders down and use your back muscles to arc your upper body upward off the ground. Pull in your abdominal muscles to avoid arching your lower back and pull your rib cage inward. Look forward and keep the back of your neck long, lifting your upper body as high as you can and keeping your shoulders stable without hunching.

3 Exhale as you move your upper body forward and down, keeping your buttocks muscles tight and lifting both legs as high as you can.

4 Continue alternating between the upper and lower body lift, 5 to 8 times each.

Variation
• **When you have enough core strength to hold your body in an arc position, as you exhale, reach your arms forward in a diving pose, keeping them forward as you inhale and rock back onto hips. To finish, place your hands on the ground in the start position and lie facedown.**

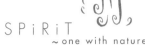

SPiRiT
~ one with nature

As you connect with your body's powerhouse, or center, and flow through the dive, feel the freedom that comes from trusting and relying on your inner strength. Connect with your own power, which is part of the power of life itself.

LISTEN TO YOUR BODY

Stop if you experience shoulder or back pain or discomfort. Practice Chest Raise (page 74) and Leg Lifts (page 75) to build strength. Do the Shell Stretch (page 99) and Cat Stretch (page 100) to stretch afterward.

BENEFITS

• Strengthens abdominal muscles, buttocks, hamstrings, and back

• Tones abdominal area, buttocks, hips, thighs, and back

• Conditions the entire back of the body

• Improves spinal mobility

• Increases self-confidence and movement control

• Enhances the mind-body connection

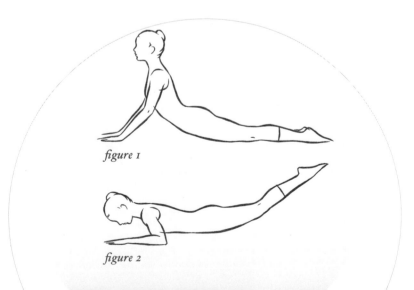

figure 1

figure 2

77

Root your hips firmly into the earth. As you extend your arms and legs, reach up and out toward opposite directions like a flower blossoming under the spring sun. Imagine opening your body's center and drawing in nourishing energy. Feel strength and peace flood your body as you flow through the movement.

LISTEN TO YOUR BODY

Avoid arching your lower back. Keep one or both feet on the ground if you cannot stabilize your pelvis. (See Double Leg Stretch I, page 60.) If you feel neck or shoulder pain or discomfort, keep upper body on the ground. Do the Full-Length Torso Stretch (page 98) to stretch your abdominal muscles afterward.

BENEFITS

- Strengthens and tones abdominal muscles
- Conditions shoulder and pelvic stabilizer muscles
- Improves shoulder mobility
- Enhances mind-body connection and integrates entire body

Double Leg Stretch II

1 Lie on your back in Base Position (page 33) with knees bent ninety degrees, feet flat on the ground, and arms at your sides with palms down.

2 Lift both of your knees at a ninety-degree angle above hips. Exhale as you reach your hands toward your ankles and peel your head and shoulders off the ground, while you gaze down at a point just above your pubic bone.

3 Inhale. Exhale as you arc your straight arms up and overhead and extend both legs to approximately forty-five degrees.

4 Inhale as you bring your arms out and down again to the start position at sides of legs, while bending knees back to ninety degrees. Keep the upper body lifted and stationary throughout arm movements. Relax shoulders, keep abdominal muscles tight, and only reach arms as far overhead as you can while maintaining upper-body lift.

5 Repeat 5 to 10 times.

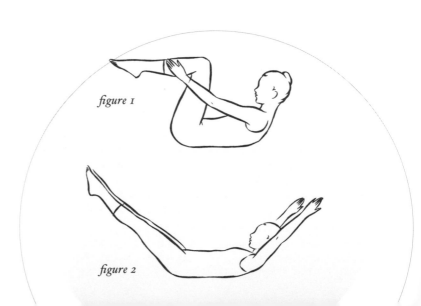

figure 1

figure 2

Leg Pull, Facing Down

1 Lie facedown, with legs straight and palms down on either side of your shoulders. Slide your shoulders down and pull in your abdominal muscles to stabilize your shoulders and back.

2 Flex toes under; exhale as you push up into a long plank, or push-up position, on the balls of your feet. Avoid locking your elbows.

3 Exhale as you lift one leg with foot flexed. Keep torso and pelvis stabilized. Do not arch your lower back. Do not drop head.

4 Inhale as you lower leg back to ball of foot.

5 Repeat with other leg.

6 Repeat, alternating legs, 3 to 10 times.

Variations
• To increase difficulty, add two or three pulses after you lift each leg to challenge your stabilizer muscles.

• For variety, alternate between flexing and pointing your foot during the pulses.

Reach deep within to feel the strength and stability in your body's center. Imagine your leg is floating up and down like a feather in the breeze. Feel your self-confidence grow from knowing and trusting in the unlimited reserves of life's power flowing through you.

LISTEN TO YOUR BODY

If you feel any wrist pain or discomfort, place a rolled towel under your palms, allowing your fingers to touch the ground. Elevating your palms relieves wrist pressure. Alternatively, perform this exercise with your elbows bent and forearms resting on the ground. To build strength for this exercise practice the Plank (page 45) and the Modified Push-Up (page 46).

BENEFITS

• Strengthens and tones shoulders, arms, buttocks, and thighs

• Conditions shoulder, spinal, and pelvic stabilizer muscles

• Improves posture

• Improves self-confidence

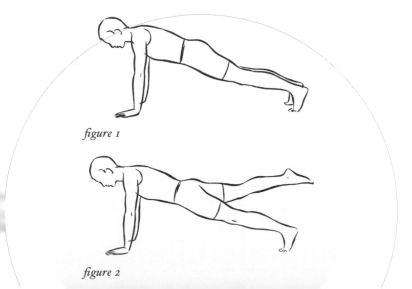

figure 1

figure 2

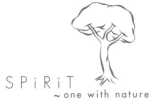

Feel strength in your lower body as you lift your center upward. Imagine yourself as a flourishing green plant reaching and growing toward the life-giving energy of the sun, and feel energized, centered, and empowered.

LISTEN TO YOUR BODY

If you feel any wrist pain or discomfort, place a rolled towel under your palms, allowing your fingers to touch the ground. Elevating your palms relieves wrist pressure. To build strength for this exercise, practice Leg Pull, Facing Up Prep (page 49), Plank (page 45), and Shoulder Bridge Prep (page 47).

BENEFITS

- Strengthens and tones shoulders, arms, buttocks, and thighs
- Conditions shoulder, spinal, and pelvic stabilizer muscles
- Stretches hamstrings
- Improves posture
- Improves self-confidence
- Enhances mind-body connection and integrates the whole body

Leg Pull, Facing Up

1 Sit with legs extended and palms down behind and outside of hips, fingers facing whatever direction is most comfortable.

2 Exhale, squeeze buttocks and hamstrings to lift your hips, and push your heels into the ground as you raise your torso upward into a plank position. With your hands under your shoulders, straighten your arms but avoid locking your elbows. Stabilize your shoulders and look straight ahead.

3 Exhale as you lift one leg as high as you can while keeping a solid plank position. Use your buttock muscles to avoid sagging at the hips. Inhale as you lower your leg, maintaining the plank position. Repeat 2 more times.

4 Repeat with the other leg. Work up to 6 repetitions on each leg.

Variation
• Lift and lower your leg 3 times before replacing your foot on the ground—first, with a pointed foot; second, with a flexed foot; and third, with a pointed foot again. Repeat with the other leg.

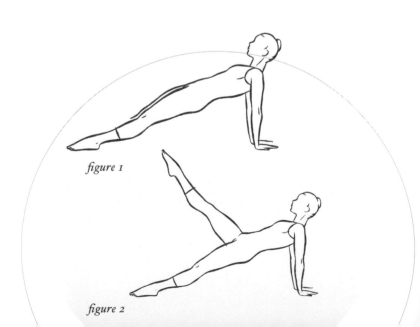

figure 1

figure 2

Swimming

1 Lie facedown, with legs extended and kneecaps touching the ground. Gently point your toes, lengthen your body, and stretch your arms out past your ears without hunching your shoulders.

2 Exhale as you pull in your abdominal muscles to establish a neutral lower back.

3 Inhale. Exhale as you raise your arms and legs to hover over the ground. Maintain your neutral lower back and lengthen your body through the back of your neck.

4 Alternate lifting one arm and the opposite leg as if you are swimming. Coordinate your breathing with the movement by inhaling for 5 beats and exhaling for 5 beats, similar to The Hundred I (page 44) breathing pattern.

5 Continue alternating arms and legs for 5 breath cycles, then lower arms and legs back to the ground.

Variations
• For an easier version, alternate lifting and lowering opposite arm and leg, but allow the nonmoving arm and leg to rest on the ground.

• To target the outer hips, rotate your legs so your heels point inward and your kneecaps face outward.

SPiRiT
~ one with nature

Imagine that you are drifting on a flowing river, taking its rushing energy into you as it carries you. Imagine that you possess the river's fluid motion and power as you breathe in and out.

LISTEN TO YOUR BODY

Avoid arching your lower back or neck. Stop if you feel lower-back or shoulder pain or discomfort. To stretch the abdominal and back muscles after this exercise, do the Shell Stretch (page 99) and Cat Stretch (page 100).

BENEFITS

• Strengthens back, buttocks, and hamstrings

• Tones shoulders, back, buttocks, hips, and thighs

• Conditions shoulder and pelvic stabilizer muscles

• Encourages lengthening of the spine, torso, arms, and legs

• Improves coordination and enhances the mind-body connection

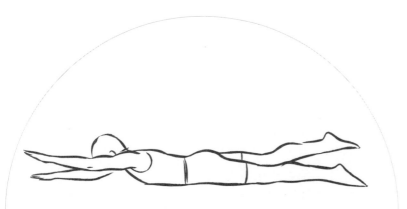

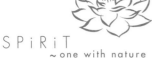

As your legs slice rhythmically through the air, connect your mind, body, and breath to experience the simplicity of the present.

LISTEN TO YOUR BODY

Do not arch your back. Stop if you are unable to stabilize your shoulders and pelvis or if you feel any neck pain or discomfort.

Modified Scissors

1 Lie on your back in Base Position (page 33) with knees bent ninety degrees, feet flat on the ground, and arms at your sides with palms down.

2 Exhale as you extend both legs toward the sky, gently pointing your toes.

3 Exhale as you curl up your upper body, reaching your arms toward your ankles.

4 Inhale as you wrap your hands around one ankle. Exhale as you lengthen the other leg by lowering it toward the ground and pulsing for 2 beats. Only lower the leg as far as you can without arching your back.

5 Inhale as you switch legs by lowering one and raising the other, switching hands to your lifted leg. Exhale as you pulse your lower leg for 2 beats.

6 Alternating legs, repeat 5 to 10 times.

7 To finish, extend both legs up toward the sky and reach your arms toward your feet. Bend and hug your knees to your chest as you lower your upper body to the ground.

Variation
• With your arms at your sides, reach toward ankles as in The Hundred I (page 44). Maintain lift and stability of upper body.

BENEFITS

- Strengthens abdominal muscles
- Tones abdominal muscles and thighs
- Stretches hamstrings and hip flexors
- Conditions shoulder and pelvic stabilizer muscles
- Invigorates and raises energy level

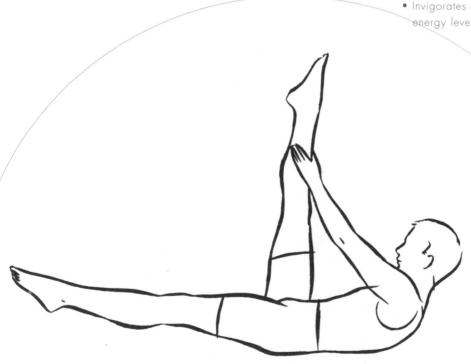

SPiRiT
~ one with nature

Working from your body's powerhouse, or center, stay mentally focused on your rhythm, balance, and control. Imagine that a gentle puff of wind is supporting you as you flow continuously and evenly.

LISTEN TO YOUR BODY

Stop if you feel lower-back pain or discomfort or have a very tight lower back. Practice Rolling Back (page 56) to increase lower-back flexibility.

Open-Leg Rocker

1 Sit on sitz (sitting) bones. Pull both of your knees toward your chest; reach toward your legs and grasp each ankle.

2 Inhale as you slide your shoulders down. Exhale and pull in your abdominal muscles as you round your spine and tilt your pelvis back so you are sitting just behind your sitz bones.

3 Inhale as you extend your legs up in a V shape slightly wider than your shoulders. Exhale as you lift your chest up, keeping your shoulders down and lengthening your spine. Look toward your ankles.

4 Inhale as you tuck your hips under and roll back onto your shoulders, lifting the sitz bones upward. Do not touch your neck or head to the ground.

5 Exhale as you contract your deep abdominal muscles and roll up to the start position.

6 Repeat 3 to 5 times.

7 To finish, bring legs together, roll upper body down, pull both of your knees toward your chest, and place your feet on the ground.

Variation
• Bend your knees ninety degrees if your legs are too tight to extend fully; hold your legs by placing your hands behind your thighs. Perform the exercise as described.

• If you cannot roll back up, simply practice balancing as you elevate and lower first one, then the other leg. finish by resting your feet back on the ground.

BENEFITS

- Strengthens deep abdominal muscles
- Stretches hamstrings
- Massages the back
- Improves coordination and concentration
- Enhances the mind-body connection

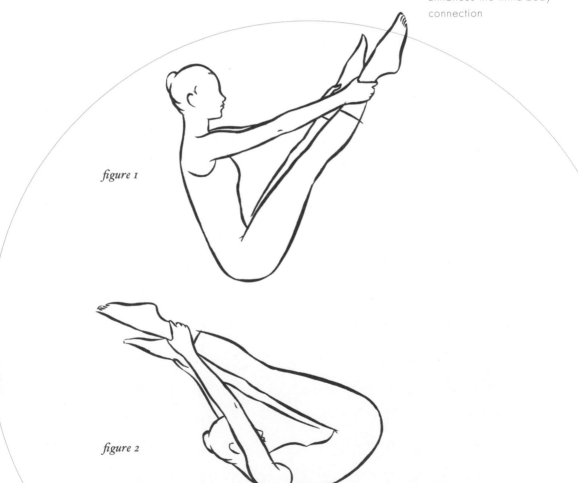

figure 1

figure 2

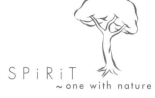

Feel the earth through your grounded foot as you press upward. Lengthen your extended leg as if to scrape the sun, connecting with the uplifting energy of the sky.

LISTEN TO YOUR BODY

Stop if you feel any back pain or discomfort. Practice Shoulder Bridge Prep (page 47) and Bridge (page 38) to build strength. Perform Knee Hug Stretch (page 96) to release any lower-back tension.

BENEFITS

* Strengthens buttocks, hamstrings, and hip flexors
* Tones buttocks, hips, thighs, and abdominal area
* Conditions spinal and pelvic stabilizer muscles
* Reinforces neutral posture
* Develops symmetry in the body for balanced muscle development

Shoulder Bridge

1 Lie on your back with a neutral spine, shoulders relaxed, arms at your sides with palms down, feet in line with hips, and knees bent less than ninety degrees as comfortable.

2 Push your feet into the ground. Exhale as you push up your torso, contracting the buttocks and hamstring muscles. Allow your weight to rest on your shoulders in the Bridge position.

3 Inhale as you lift one knee above your hip, gently point your toes, and extend your leg toward the sky, keeping stable in the Bridge position.

4 Exhale as you flex your foot, then lengthen and lower your leg until it is in line with the other thigh. Keep the Bridge position and a neutral spinal alignment. Inhale as you gently point your toes and lengthen your leg back toward the sky.

5 Repeat 3 times.

6 Bend your knee and place your foot on the ground.

7 Repeat with the opposite leg.

8 To finish, lower your hips to the ground.

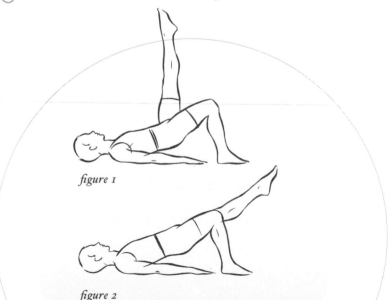

figure 1

figure 2

Saw

1 Sit with neutral spinal alignment, legs extended and spread slightly wider than your hips. Flex your feet, pull in your abdominal muscles, relax your shoulders, and place your hands next to your hips. If your pelvis tilts backward, wedge a rolled towel under it to tilt it forward into a neutral position.

2 Exhale as you reach your arms out wide toward opposite directions, keeping your shoulders relaxed. Inhale as you lengthen your spine from the top of your head, lifting your ribs away from your hips and lengthening your waist, while keeping your pelvis grounded. Feel a sense of openness and lightness between each vertebra in the spine.

3 Exhale as you rotate at the waist and dive forward headfirst, reaching your left arm toward your right leg. Pull in your abdominal muscles and reach your pinkie finger past your small toe as if you are going to saw it. Stabilize your shoulders and reach your back arm behind you.

4 Inhale as you roll up, stacking each vertebra like building blocks. Return to center in a neutral posture and extend your arms out to the sides again.

5 Alternating sides, repeat 5 to 10 times.

Variation
• If the backs of your legs are tight, bend your knees slightly.

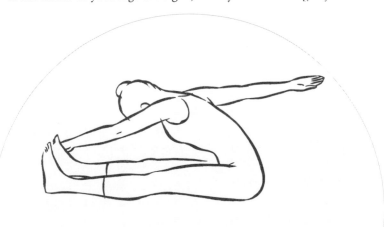

SPiRiT
~ one with nature

Root your hips firmly into the ground, drawing on the earth's stability. Feel energy rolling through your spine like waves. Imagine waves of energy cascading across your body out through your fingertips, as you dive down and reach out, twisting and extending yourself to reach new shores. Enjoy the expansive energy from stretching and opening going to places you have not been before.

LISTEN TO YOUR BODY

Stop if you cannot rotate your spine without lifting your sitz (sitting) bones. Practice Spine Stretch (page 62), Spine Twist (page 64), and Circle Shoulder, Chest, and Back Stretch (page 102) to increase your flexibility.

BENEFITS

• Opens up chest and straightens rounded shoulders

• Improves spinal mobility

• Conditions pelvic and shoulder stabilizer muscles

• Stretches the back, especially the lower back, hamstrings, and waist

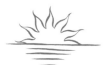

Teaser

1 Lie on your back in Base Position (page 33) with knees bent ninety degrees, feet flat on the ground, and arms at your sides with palms down.

2 Exhale as you lift one, then the other knee above your hips. Inhale. As you exhale, extend both legs toward the sky, gently pointing your toes. Arc both arms up and over your head past your ears, keeping your rib cage grounded.

3 Inhale as you start lifting your arms up toward sky. Exhale as you peel spine up, one vertebra at a time, while lowering legs until you make a V shape with your torso and legs. Sit just behind your sitz (sitting) bones with arms extended parallel to legs.

4 Inhale as you hold the position.

5 Exhale as you roll down, one vertebra at a time, lowering your arms as you lower your spine toward the ground and keep your legs elevated.

6 Repeat 3 to 5 times.

7 To finish, roll your upper body down. Hug your knees to the chest to stretch your lower back.

Variation
• For an easier version, keep one knee bent and one foot on the ground during the exercise. Do the first half of your repetitions lifting only one leg. Switch legs and do the remaining repetitions.

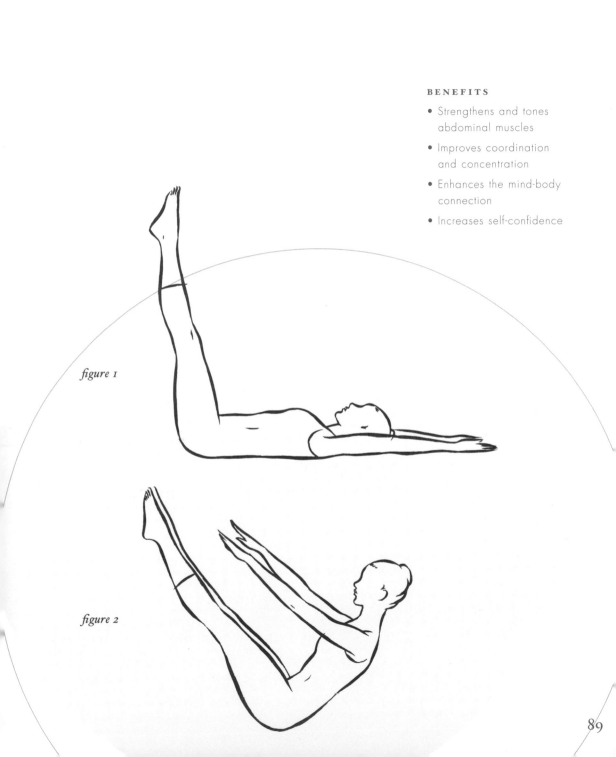

BENEFITS

- Strengthens and tones abdominal muscles
- Improves coordination and concentration
- Enhances the mind-body connection
- Increases self-confidence

figure 1

figure 2

89

sitting quietly,
doing nothing,
spring comes,
and the grass
grows by
itself.

{Zen saying}

In our fast-paced society, we tend to value motion, energy,
and productivity. Often this attitude leads to mental and
physical overload and we find ourselves feeling run-
down, tense, and stressed out. Eastern philosophers
hold that tension and stiffness can eventually lead to
disease. For optimum health, we need to release our
tension and restore balance in our bodies and minds. We
can accomplish this by focusing and relaxing our minds,
monitoring our breathing, and stretching our bodies.

Stretching provides a release of muscular tension.
Relaxing the mind through use of imagery and visualization helps to release mental tension. Breathing exercises complement relaxation exercises by connecting
the mind and body and helping you to be aware of the
present. All of these practices—stretching, relaxation,
and breathing—strengthen your mental fitness and
encourage physical flexibility.

In the East, a relaxed and supple body is believed
to reflect ideal health. Physical tension denotes an
imbalance or blockage in the flow of life-force energy.
Through regular practice of your exercises, your awareness of muscular tension increases. Regular stretching
and movement enables you to begin releasing excess
muscular tension to restore healthy muscle tone.
Circulation of blood (as well as life-force energy)
improves, bringing nutrients to formerly undernourished

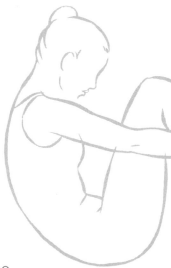

areas of the body. **Movement and health are restored to previously underused areas of your body. You dramatically increase your use of your body to maintain optimum vigor and health.**

Stretches

Traditionally, Pilates exercises did not focus on stretches. Our modern lifestyle, however, contributes to muscular tension and stiffness for many people. Stretching can release this tension, enhance feelings of well-being, and prevent cramping and muscle exhaustion during long workouts. The stretches that follow do all this, in addition to effectively counterbalancing your Pilates exercises.

Stretching is a "feel good" activity and should never be performed if it causes you any pain. Hold each stretch to a point of moderate tension, and make sure the tension is felt in your muscles, not in your joints. Hold each stretch for 15 to 30 seconds. Hold the stretch position during inhalation and increase the stretch and release tension with each exhalation.

The Power of Combining Stretches with Visualization

Exercises that involve focusing on mental imagery to enhance relaxation are becoming increasingly widespread. Many hospitals now use guided imagery exercises with patients before and after surgical procedures to reduce stress and promote healing. Some cancer patients also use imagery to make chemotherapy less unpleasant. The "Spirit—One with Nature" cues in this chapter provide visualizations that you can use to help release your muscular tension and feelings of stress.

During each stretch, as you focus on releasing tightness and tension from your muscles, concentrate on allowing stress to drain away from your mind. Use your exercise time as an opportunity to harmonize your movements with your internal

BELLY BREATHING

Diaphragmatic belly breathing stimulates the relaxation response and helps bring your body back into balance after experiencing and responding to stress. Each time you perform any of your stretching exercises, make an effort to breathe deeply. In this manner, you can maximize their relaxation effect and condition your respiratory muscles.

The belly breathing exercise technique below can be used during your stretches. This technique differs from the expansive rib cage style of breathing that characterizes your Pilates exercises.

1 Sit or lie comfortably. Place your hands on your belly to increase your awareness of its movement.

2 Inhale fully, keeping your shoulders soft and relaxed, as you feel the expansion in your belly.

3 Exhale fully, as you notice your belly moving inward.

4 Breathe deeply for 1 minute.

5 Notice your mental state. Do you feel more relaxed?

This belly breathing exercise can help you develop a more relaxed, diaphragmatic breathing pattern. Do not be surprised if at first you are so accustomed to holding in your abdominals that you find it difficult to relax and allow your belly to expand. With focused practice you can relearn to breathe naturally.

Progressive relaxation is an effective technique to increase your awareness of tightness in your body. Before you can consciously release tension from your muscles, you need to know what muscle tension in your body feels like. You can practice progressive relaxation at your desk during a break or in bed before you fall asleep at night.

1 Sit or lie comfortably.

2 Tighten all the muscles in your head: squint your eyes, clench your teeth, and tighten your scalp.

3 Inhale fully through your nose. Exhale through your nose, relaxing all the muscles in your head. Soften the muscles around your hairline, allow your eyes to sink deeply into your head, soften your throat, and relax your jaw. Open your mouth and throat wide as if you are yawning and really stretch your face.

4 Allow all the muscles in your head to remain relaxed.

5 Contract and release each of the major muscle groups in your body one by one, from the top of your head to the tips of your toes. Relax your entire body.

continued on page 93

sense of well-being. Awaken your senses to the beauty of the natural world and align your perspective to feel your place in nature. When you do so, each exercise session will leave you feeling refreshed, replenished, and relaxed.

Benefits of Deep Breathing

Breath is the link between your body and mind—an unconscious process that can be made conscious. In many ancient cultures, breath is laden with spiritual implications since breathing is our first act when we are born and our last when we pass away. Breath, therefore, is a powerful affirmation of life.

Deep-breathing exercises can give both physical and emotional benefits. Research shows that deep, diaphragmatic breathing practices can reduce blood pressure, heart rate, and feelings of anxiety. In addition, the action of the lungs, diaphragm, and thorax pumps lymphatic fluids throughout the body, supporting the immune system.

If you don't have time for a full or even abbreviated Pilates workout session, simply take a few moments during your day to observe your breathing. Pay particular attention to how the breath moves your body, noticing subtleties, such as whether your chest or belly rises with inhalation, and how your body responds to exhalation. This singular focus brings you into the present moment and into the immediate experience of your body. Simply observing your breath often results in slower, deeper diaphragmatic breaths that further relax your body.

Deep within each of us lies a well of peaceful calm. By doing visualization exercises, breathing from your belly, and stretching your muscles, you can use your exercise time to connect with this inner serenity. Celebrate the joy of movement, the striking beauty of life itself, and your inner self. You will feel relaxed, refreshed, and energetic.

Stress

Stress is an inevitable part of modern life, and it manifests in several different ways. Physical and mental signs include:

- increased blood pressure
- increased heart rate
- increased blood flow to the extremities
- reduced blood flow to digestive organs
- increased blood cortisol levels
- increased perspiration
- muscle tension
- anxiety
- mental tension
- hyperalertness

These symptoms appear when we experience more stress than our bodies can handle and we do not discharge the resulting tension. The body is not designed to live in chronic stress. Long-term stress can affect our physical and mental health, making us more susceptible to illness, depression, and anxiety disorders. Therefore, we need to release our tensions before they start to build up. Unfortunately, since many stress-causing situations do not require physical responses (like running away from a predator) we do not have a natural way to "burn off" the stress response. Consequently, we need to implement alternative measures such as breathing and relaxation exercises to return the body and mind to a calm, balanced state.

Benefits of Stretching

The idea that stretching is healthy and beneficial may seem obvious, but in our busy lives it can be easy to neglect this aspect of our exercise routines. To help you remember to stretch before and after working out, and even when you're just feeling tense, below are the benefits of stretching the body.

6 Inhale fully through your nose and simultaneously tighten every muscle in your body: clench your fists, squeeze your heels together, tighten your buttocks, grit your teeth, and make every other muscle tight, tight, tight.

7 Exhale powerfully, releasing all the tension in your body. Gently rock your body. Take a big yawn and do a leisurely full-body stretch like a cat waking up from a long nap in the morning sun.

8 Enjoy this feeling of complete relaxation.

9 Repeat as needed.

"STRAW" OR PURSED-LIP BREATHING EXERCISE

This exercise increases your awareness of diaphragmatic breathing, helps you to increase the length and depth of your exhalation, and helps you avoid shallow "overbreathing."

You will need a drinking straw for this exercise.

1 Inhale through your nose.

2 Make a long slow exhalation through the straw.

3 Count your breath cycles for one minute. (One inhalation and one exhalation equal one breath cycle.)

Notice how you feel during the experience. Explore any emotional reactions, such as fear of not drawing in enough air or impatience over exhaling slowly. Practicing this exercise will help you gradually become more comfortable and patient with slower breathing. It will also improve your ability to take longer, slower exhalations. An ideal rate of relaxed breathing is six breath cycles per minute.

STRETCHING

- increases your ability to move fully and freely
- improves your balance
- encourages balanced muscle development, which increases joint stability
- reduces your risk of injury and muscle soreness
- improves your posture
- prevents lower back pain
- alleviates muscle cramps
- improves joint health by lubricating joints when taken through a full range of motion
- improves athletic performance
- enhances strength-training results by preventing feelings of tightness or stiffness
- releases muscle tension and helps you relax

Rules for Static Stretches

- Move slowly to the edge of your range of motion.
- Concentrate on the muscle being stretched.
- Exhale, relax, and allow your muscle to release gradually; inhale and check your alignment.
- Start with a fifteen-second stretch, work up to twenty or thirty seconds.
- Always move deliberately, with control.
- Always feel the stretch in the central area of the muscle.
- If you feel any pain or tightness in your joint, ease up on the stretch. Pain in your joints means you are stretching too hard.
- Stretch during and after every training session.
- Do NOT bounce.
- Do NOT move quickly.
- NEVER apply force.
- Do NOT lock your joints.
- Do NOT go beyond a joint's natural range of motion or hyperextend your joints.
- Do NOT stretch an injured joint.
- Do NOT stretch a torn muscle.

Knee Sways Stretch

1 Lie on your back in Base Position (page 33) with knees bent ninety degrees, feet flat on the ground, and arms slightly away from sides in an A shape with palms up.

2 Pull your knees and feet together.

3 Inhale. Exhale as you allow both legs to fall to the left side and your right hip to lift off the ground, keeping your shoulder blades on the ground and your knees bent. Feel the stretch along the side of your torso and in your lower back.

4 Inhale as you pull your legs and hips back to the center position.

5 Repeat, dropping your legs to the right side.

6 Alternating sides, repeat 5 to 10 times.

Variation
• **After completing at least 3 repetitions on each side, you may hold your knees to one side for a static stretch for one or two breath cycles. (One inhalation and one exhalation equal one breath cycle.) Repeat on the other side.**

SPiRiT
~ one with nature

Imagine that the earth beneath you is an absorbent sponge. As you release your breath, allow any stressful feelings stored in your back to drain into the sponge. As you inhale, feel the lightness that fills your body after you have let go of stress and tension. Continue releasing tension with each exhalation.

BENEFITS

• Improves spinal mobility

• Releases tension from the middle and lower back

• Stretches the lower back, waist, and hips

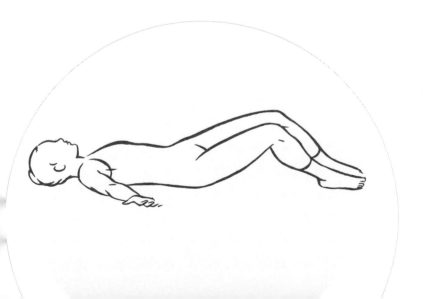

Feel the nurturing comfort of
the earth beneath you. As you
exhale, allow any tension in
your back or buttocks to melt
away like a snowflake in
warm water. With each
inhalation, draw in new energy.

LISTEN TO YOUR BODY

You should not feel any pain.
Relax, breathe, and ease
gently into this stretch.

BENEFITS

- Stretches lower back,
  buttocks, and inner thighs
- Releases tension from lower
  back and hips

Knee Hug Stretch

1 Lie on your back in Base Position (page 33) with knees bent
ninety degrees, feet flat on the ground, and arms at your sides with
palms down.

2 Place your arms around the backs of your thighs. Pull both
knees toward your chest. Avoid putting any pressure on your
knees. Inhale as you hold the position.

3 Exhale as you gently pull your knees closer toward your chest.
Feel the stretch in your buttocks and lower back. Hold for 15 to
30 seconds.

Variations

- For an inner-thigh stretch, pull your knees toward your shoulders.
Feel the stretch in your inner thighs, buttocks, and lower back. Hold
for 15 to 30 seconds.

- For a lower-back massage, gently circle legs together, feeling the
movement in your lower back and hips and at the base of your spine.

- For a seated variation, sit comfortably in your chair with both feet flat
on the ground. Place your arms around the back of one thigh. As you
exhale, draw your knee toward your chest, keeping your other foot on
the ground. Continue breathing, focusing on the exhalation as you feel
the stretch in your buttocks and lower back. Hold for 15 to 30 seconds.

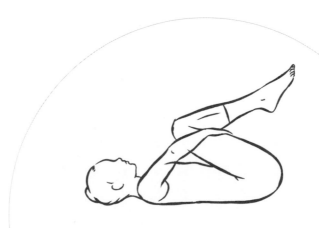

Neck Stretch

1 Lie on your back in Base Position (page 33) with your knees bent ninety degrees, feet flat on the ground, and arms at your sides with palms down. Reach overhead, placing your palms on the back of your head, with elbows up.

2 Inhale. Exhale as you lift your chin toward your chest, supporting your head with your hands. Look down the front of your torso, keeping your shoulders relaxed. Relax the weight of your head into hands. Feel the stretch behind the central part of your neck. Do not compress chin into chest.

3 Hold for 3 breath cycles. (One inhalation and one exhalation equal one breath cycle.)

4 Inhale. Exhale as you lower head to ground.

Variation

• For a seated variation, sit comfortably in your chair and place your hands on the back of your head. Allow your chin to drop toward your chest, keeping your shoulders relaxed. Do not pull on your head or compress chin into chest. Feel a gentle stretch behind the central part of your neck. Lift your head back to normal position. Return your arms to your sides.

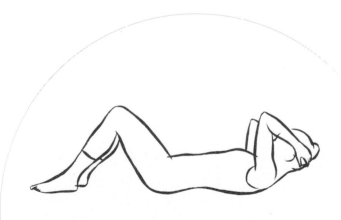

SPiRiT
~ one with nature

As you exhale, shed any worries that are stored in your neck and shoulders. Allow stresses to drain down into the absorbent earth below you as you relax your breath, body, and mind. Imagine your heart and mind opening up like the petals of a flower. Enjoy the fresh feeling of lightness as you let go of your tensions.

LISTEN TO YOUR BODY

Stretch your neck gently and without pain. Release from the stretch slowly.

BENEFITS

• Improves neck mobility
• Encourages lengthening of neck
• Releases tension from neck and shoulders

Imagine a glowing ball of light at your body's center. As you stretch, let light stream throughout your body as you extend your fingertips and toes to opposite horizons, illuminating and refreshing you.

BENEFITS

- Stretches the entire torso, particularly the waist
- Releases tension throughout the body

Full-Length Torso Stretch

1 Lie on your back in Base Position (page 33) with knees bent ninety degrees, feet flat on the ground, and arms at your sides with palms down.

2 Extend and straighten your legs. Extend your arms overhead past your ears.

3 Inhale. Exhale as you reach the arm and leg on one side of your body toward opposite directions and lengthen your waist by drawing your rib cage away from your pelvis. Continue to breathe normally as you hold the stretch for 15 to 30 seconds.

4 Repeat on other side.

5 From your center, lengthen both arms and both legs together, stretching in opposite directions. If comfortable, arch your rib cage up to increase your torso stretch.

Variation

• For a seated variation, sit comfortably in your chair with your shoulders relaxed, feet placed on the ground hip-width apart, and arms at your sides with palms in. Hold the side of the chair with one hand. Exhale as you lift your other arm palm up in a long arc out to the side and over your head. Feel the stretch in the side of your torso. Continue to breathe normally as you hold the stretch for 15 to 30 seconds. Bring your arm down in an arc out to the side. Repeat on other side.

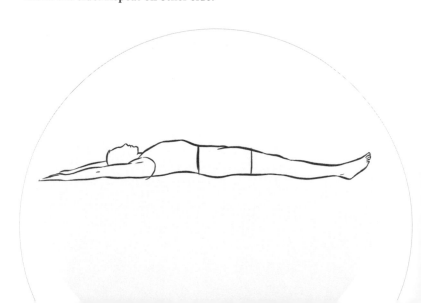

Shell Stretch

1 Kneel on all fours with your hands under your shoulders and your knees under your hips, in a "table" position.

2 Exhale and lift your abdominal muscles as you tuck in your tailbone and lower your hips toward your heels as far as is comfortable for your knees. With palms on the ground, lengthen your arms. Continue to breathe, focusing on expanding your rib cage with each inhalation and rounding your lower back with each exhalation. Hold for 15 to 30 seconds.

3 To finish, lift hips back up to start position.

SPiRiT
~ one with nature

Imagine that your back is a sun-bathing tortoise's shell. Inhale up and into your shell, feeling safe and comfortable. As you exhale, feel the warmth of the sun on your back melting any tensions and allow them to drain into the ground. Enjoy the nurturing, stable support of the earth beneath you. Continue to relax your mind and body, releasing unneeded thoughts, worries, and stresses.

LISTEN TO YOUR BODY

If you have any knee pain or discomfort, do not lower your hips completely to your heels. If this modification does not help, substitute the Knee Hug Stretch (page 96).

BENEFITS

- Stretches the back, shoulders, and rib cage
- Releases tension throughout the body

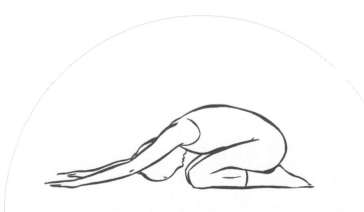

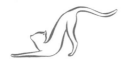

All natural life is filled with rhythm and motion. Imagine that you are as supple and graceful as a purring cat. Use your suppleness to flow naturally and rhythmically with the pulse of life, through your spine and with your breath.

LISTEN TO YOUR BODY

If your knees are not comfortable in a table position, substitute the Knee Hug Stretch (page 96).

BENEFITS

- Improves spinal mobility
- Stretches the back
- Increases body awareness
- Enhances the mind-body connection

Cat Stretch

1 Kneel on all fours with hands under shoulders and knees under hips, in a "table" position. Maintain neutral spinal alignment and lengthen through neck and torso.

2 Exhale as you round your spine by tucking in the tailbone. Spread shoulder blades wide and allow neck to relax by dropping head.

3 Inhale as you return to start position.

4 Repeat 5 to 10 times. Flow through motion without stopping, feeling fluidity and suppleness in your spine.

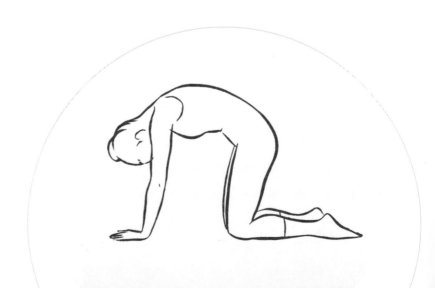

Deep Buttocks Stretch

1 Lie on your back in Base Position (page 33) with your knees bent ninety degrees, feet flat on the ground, and arms at your sides with palms down.

2 Pull your right knee toward your chest, place your right ankle on top of your left thigh, and place both hands around the back of your left thigh. Inhale.

3 Exhale as you pull your left thigh toward your chest. Continue breathing, lengthening the stretch with each exhalation. Hold stretch for 15 to 30 seconds.

4 Inhale. Exhale as you unwrap legs and return to start position.

5 Repeat with other leg.

SPiRiT
~ one with nature

With each exhalation, imagine letting your tensions soak deep into the ground beneath you. Imagine this stream flowing far into the absorbent earth, carrying away your cares and burdens. Surrender to gravity.

BENEFITS

- Stretches the deep buttocks muscles
- Releases tension from the lower back and hips
- Improves hip flexibility
- Helps prevent sciatica

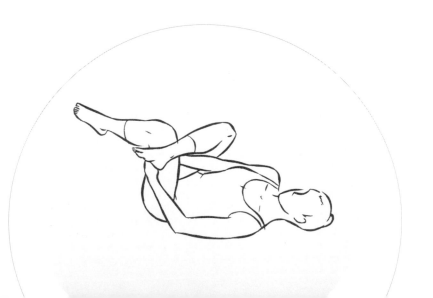

Imagine you are creating a circle of protective light with each sweep of your arm. Inhale as you draw in healing, restorative energy to bathe every cell in your body. Exhale as you release unneeded tension. As you open your chest and shoulders, open your heart to receive all the goodness and richness in your life.

LISTEN TO YOUR BODY

Stop if you feel any shoulder pain or discomfort.

Circle Shoulder, Chest, and Back Stretch

1 Lie on your back in Base Position (page 33) with knees bent ninety degrees, feet flat on the ground, and arms at your sides with palms down.

2 Slide left heel down.

3 Rotate your waist to the left and drop your right knee across your body as you place the left hand on the outside of the right leg. Extend your right arm in the opposite direction.

4 Turn your head to look at your right hand. Rotate your right palm upward. Drag your knuckles or fingers in a semicircle on the ground as if making a "snow angel." Repeat 3 to 5 times.

5 To finish, position your arm directly out to the side. Roll onto your back, hugging the knees toward your chest and stretching your lower back and buttocks. Return to the start position, placing your feet flat on the ground with bent knees.

6 Repeat on the other side.

Variation
• To further open up and stretch your back, instead of rolling onto your back after making the snow-angel motion remain in the twist with arms extended wide in a T position. Sweep your right arm across the sky in an arc and touch your left palm. Tuck your chin toward your chest, stretching the back of your neck. Direct your breath into your upper back. Feel the stretch in the middle of your upper back between your shoulder blades. Hold the stretch for 15 to 30 seconds. Roll onto your back and continue the exercise. Repeat variation on the other side.

BENEFITS

- Stretches the chest, shoulder, torso, and hip muscles

- Releases tension from the chest, shoulders, middle and lower back, and hips

- Improves spinal mobility

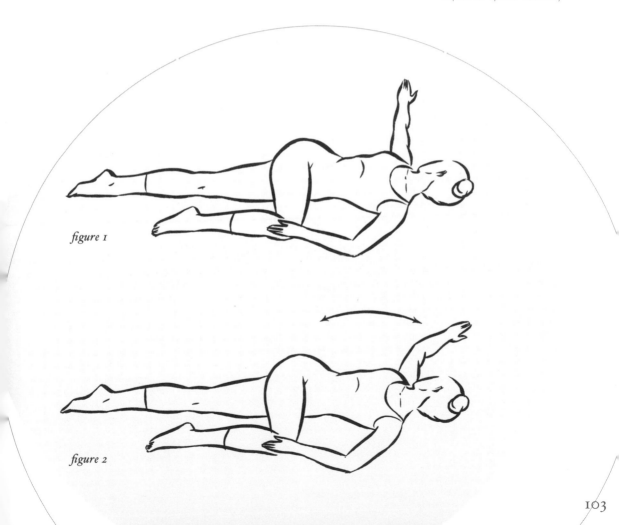

figure 1

figure 2

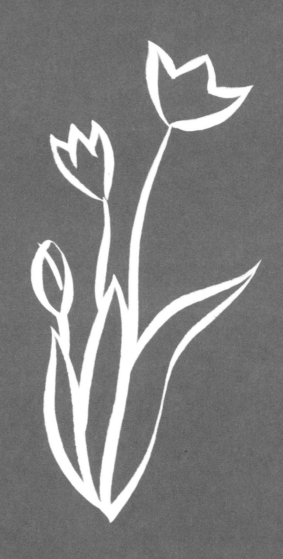

part III

MAKING PILATES FUSION A
PaRT OF YOUR LIFE

Flow with whatever may happen and let your mind be free.
Stay centered by accepting whatever you are doing.
This is the ultimate.

{Chuang Tsu}

> If I had
> two loaves of
> bread, I would
> sell one and buy
> hyacinths, for
> they would
> feed my soul.
>
> {The Koran}

chapter 7

RouTiNeS:
PUTTING IT ALL TOGETHER

Now that you're comfortable doing the exercises, it's time to pull them together into routines that fit your specific needs. Whether you have fifteen minutes or an entire hour, you'll find a sequence here for you. I've ordered the routines from beginning to advanced. The beginning routines are great for those who are new to the practice or for veterans looking for a gentler exercise session. The more advanced routines challenge your strength, flexibility, and coordination.

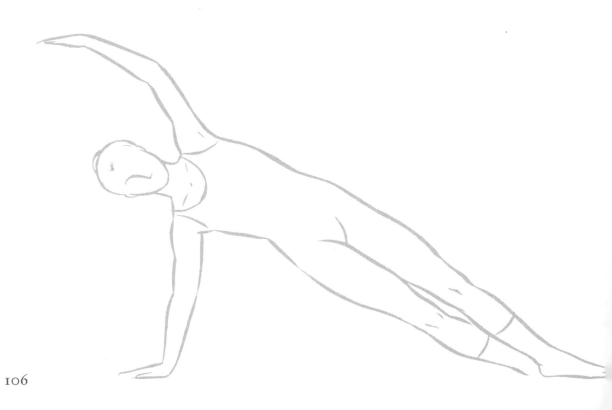

Ideally, you'll perform a forty-five-minute to one-hour routine at least two or three times a week. If you can, squeeze in a short routine or a stretching and breathing workout on the other days to further your progress. Remember that any physical activity you do is better than doing nothing. Everyone has time to breathe, so at the very least squeeze in a breathing exercise every day.

The following exercise routines are presented with sequential thumbnail illustrations for easy reference.

- Good Morning Wake-Up Routine (15 minutes)
- Workday Survival Routine (15 minutes)
- Back and Lower-Body Relaxation Stretch Routine (5 minutes)
- Busy Day Strong and Stretched Routine (20 minutes)
- Basic Full-Body Workout (45 minutes)
- Intermediate Full-Body Workout (45 minutes)
- Advanced Full-Body Workout (60 minutes)
- Total Body Relaxation Stretch Routine (25 minutes)
- Nighttime Wind-Down Routine (15 minutes)

Try to do the Basic Full-Body Routine at least two or three times a week. When you are short on time, practice the Good Morning Wake-Up Routine. If you have a few more minutes to practice, combine this with the Nighttime Wind-Down Routine. If you work in an office or other stress-filled environment, squeeze in the Workday Survival Routine whenever possible.

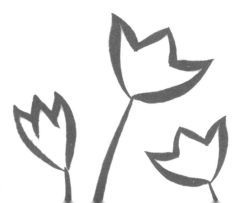

As your strength, flexibility, and coordination improve, switch from the Basic Full-Body Routine to the Intermediate Full-Body Workout and then to the Advanced Full-Body Workout. When moving from the Basic to the Intermediate workout, you can start out by doing the Basic routine twice a week and the Intermediate routine once a week, increasing the challenge gradually as is comfortable for your body.

On days when you're too tired to exercise, simply try to fit in a stretching routine or a progressive relaxation or breathing exercise. This will keep your body in a conditioning mode, which will enhance your practice the next time you work out. The short stretching routines listed above can also be used by advanced exercisers on low-energy days or for an occasional body-awareness check-in.

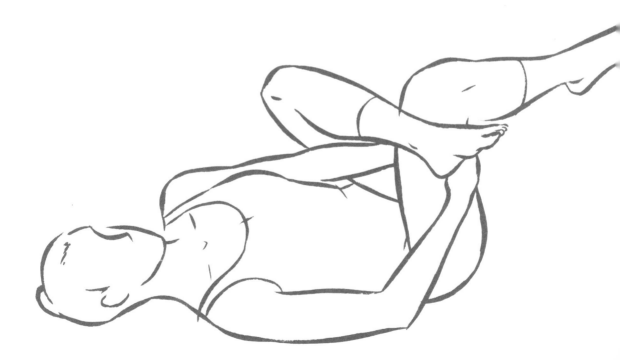

GooD MoRNiNG
WAKE-UP ROUTINE

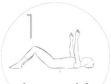

base position
(page 33)

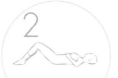

pilates breathing
(page 34)

pelvic tilt
(page 36)

bridge
(page 38)

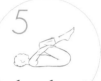

knee hug stretch
(page 96)

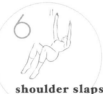

shoulder slaps
(page 39)

bridge *(page 38)*,
rib cage arms
(page 40)

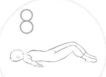

knee sways stretch
(page 95)

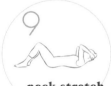

neck stretch
(page 97)

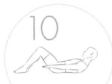

**curl-up
with long arms**
(page 43)

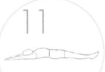

**full-length
torso stretch**
(page 98)

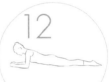

plank
(page 45)

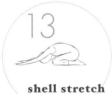

shell stretch
(page 99)

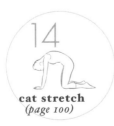

cat stretch
(page 100)

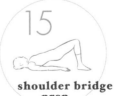

**shoulder bridge
prep**
(page 47)

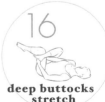

**deep buttocks
stretch**
(page 101)

roll-up
(page 54)

rolling back
(page 56)

WoRKDay
SURVIVAL ROUTINE

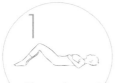

1

**pilates breathing,
seated**
(page 34)

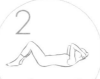

2

neck stretch
(page 97)

3

**knee hug stretch,
seated**
(page 96)

4

spine twist
(page 64)

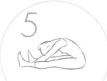

5

spine stretch
(page 62)

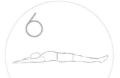

6

**full-length torso
stretch, seated**
(page 98)

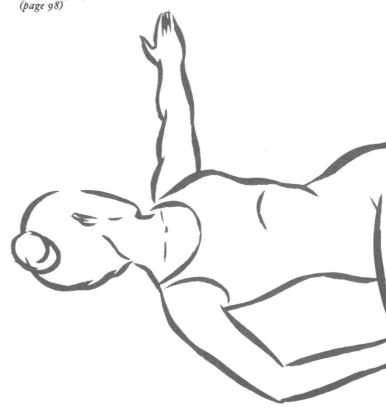

BaCK aND LoWeR-BoDY
RELAXATION STRETCH ROUTINE

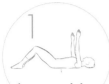

1

base position
(page 33)

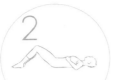

2

pilates breathing
(page 34)

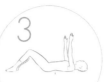

3

pelvic tilt
(page 36)

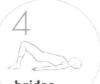

4

bridge
(page 38)

5

knee hug stretch
(page 96)

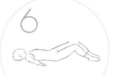

6

knee sways stretch
(page 95)

7

**deep buttocks
stretch**
(page 101)

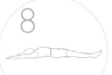

8

**full-length
torso stretch**
(page 98)

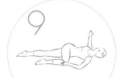

9

**circle shoulder, chest,
and back stretch**
(page 102)

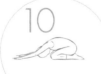

10

shell stretch
(page 99)

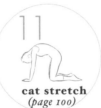

11

cat stretch
(page 100)

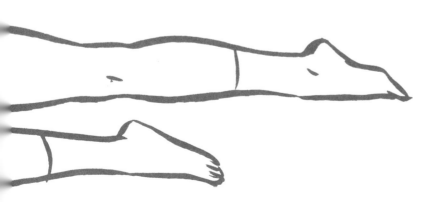

BuSY DaY
STRONG AND STRETCHED ROUTINE

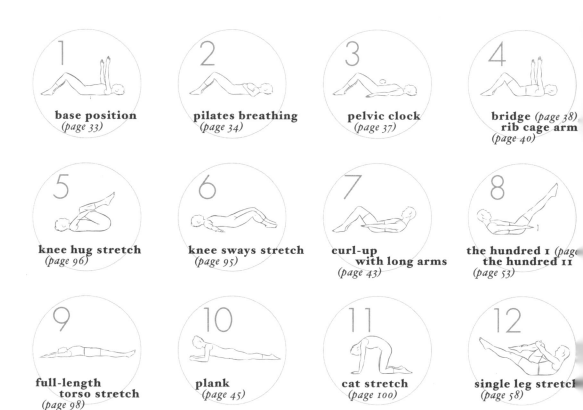

1 base position
(page 33)

2 pilates breathing
(page 34)

3 pelvic clock
(page 37)

4 bridge *(page 38)*
rib cage arm
(page 40)

5 knee hug stretch
(page 96)

6 knee sways stretch
(page 95)

7 curl-up
with long arms
(page 43)

8 the hundred I *(page*
the hundred II
(page 53)

9 full-length
torso stretch
(page 98)

10 plank
(page 45)

11 cat stretch
(page 100)

12 single leg stretch
(page 58)

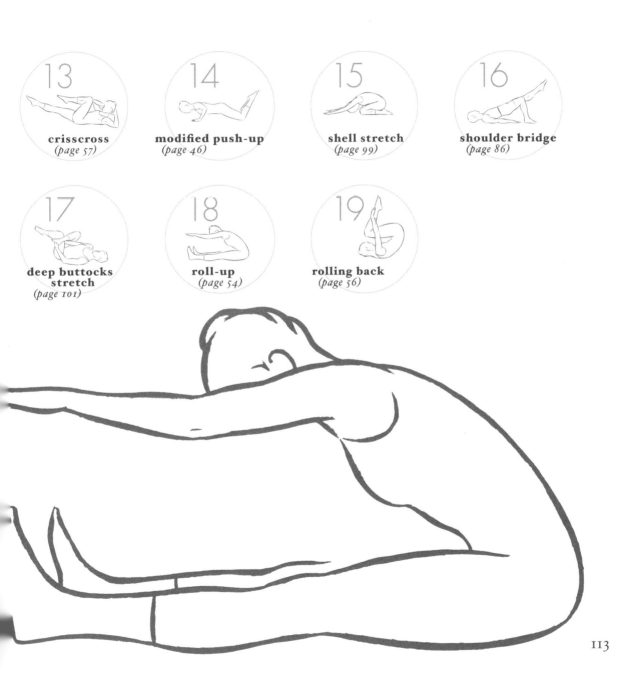

13 crisscross
(page 57)

14 modified push-up
(page 46)

15 shell stretch
(page 99)

16 shoulder bridge
(page 86)

17 deep buttocks stretch
(page 101)

18 roll-up
(page 54)

19 rolling back
(page 56)

BaSiC
FULL-BODY WORKOUT

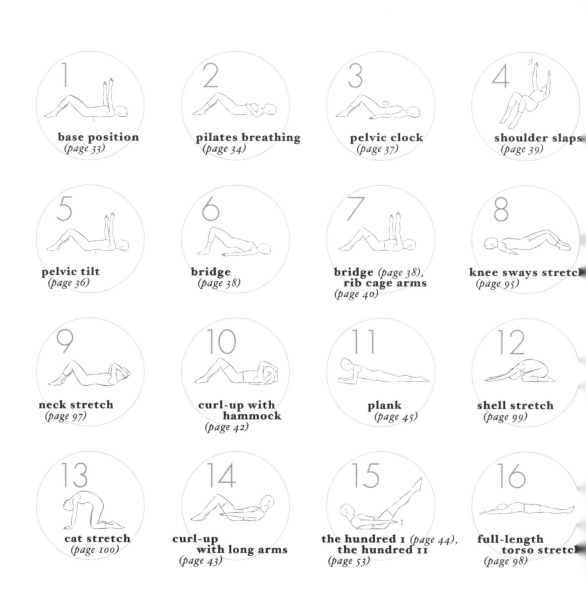

1 base position
(page 33)

2 pilates breathing
(page 34)

3 pelvic clock
(page 37)

4 shoulder slaps
(page 39)

5 pelvic tilt
(page 36)

6 bridge
(page 38)

7 bridge *(page 38)*,
rib cage arms
(page 40)

8 knee sways stretch
(page 95)

9 neck stretch
(page 97)

10 curl-up with
hammock
(page 42)

11 plank
(page 45)

12 shell stretch
(page 99)

13 cat stretch
(page 100)

14 curl-up
with long arms
(page 43)

15 the hundred I *(page 44)*,
the hundred II
(page 53)

16 full-length
torso stretch
(page 98)

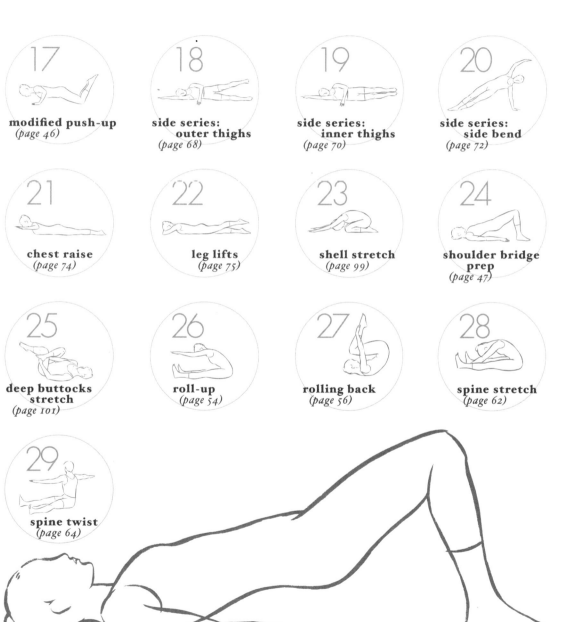

17 modified push-up
(page 46)

18 side series:
    outer thighs
(page 68)

19 side series:
    inner thighs
(page 70)

20 side series:
    side bend
(page 72)

21 chest raise
(page 74)

22 leg lifts
(page 75)

23 shell stretch
(page 99)

24 shoulder bridge
prep
(page 47)

25 deep buttocks
stretch
(page 101)

26 roll-up
(page 54)

27 rolling back
(page 56)

28 spine stretch
(page 62)

29 spine twist
(page 64)

iNTeRMeDiaTe
FULL-BODY WORKOUT

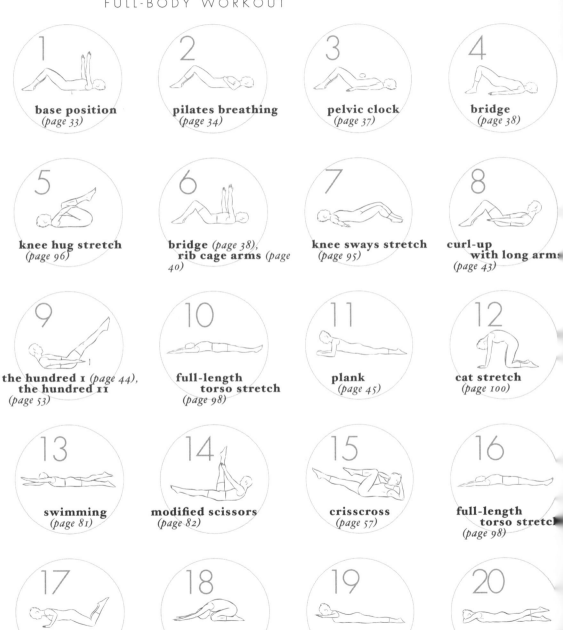

1 **base position** *(page 33)*

2 **pilates breathing** *(page 34)*

3 **pelvic clock** *(page 37)*

4 **bridge** *(page 38)*

5 **knee hug stretch** *(page 96)*

6 **bridge** *(page 38),* **rib cage arms** *(page 40)*

7 **knee sways stretch** *(page 95)*

8 **curl-up with long arms** *(page 43)*

9 **the hundred I** *(page 44),* **the hundred II** *(page 53)*

10 **full-length torso stretch** *(page 98)*

11 **plank** *(page 45)*

12 **cat stretch** *(page 100)*

13 **swimming** *(page 81)*

14 **modified scissors** *(page 82)*

15 **crisscross** *(page 57)*

16 **full-length torso stretch** *(page 98)*

17 **modified push-up** *(page 46)*

18 **shell stretch** *(page 99)*

19 **chest raise** *(page 74)*

20 **leg lifts** *(page 75)*

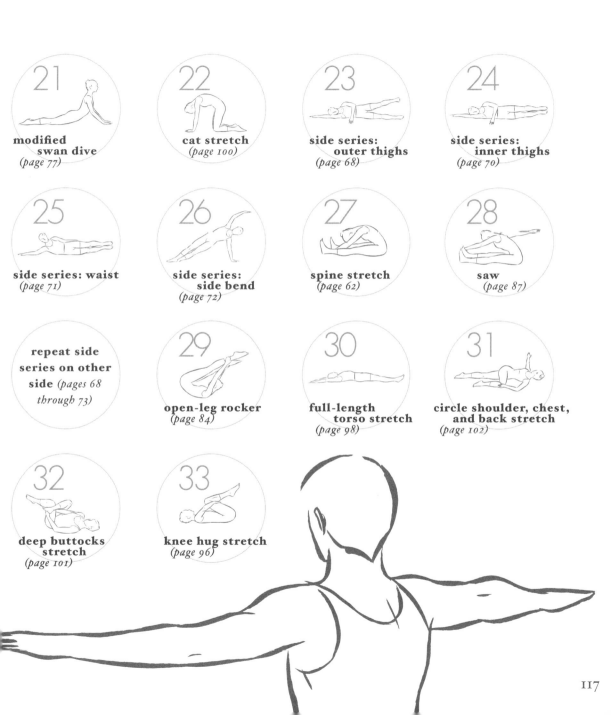

21 modified
swan dive
(page 77)

22 cat stretch
(page 100)

23 side series:
outer thighs
(page 68)

24 side series:
inner thighs
(page 70)

25 side series: waist
(page 71)

26 side series:
side bend
(page 72)

27 spine stretch
(page 62)

28 saw
(page 87)

repeat side
series on other
side *(pages 68
through 73)*

29 open-leg rocker
(page 84)

30 full-length
torso stretch
(page 98)

31 circle shoulder, chest,
and back stretch
(page 102)

32 deep buttocks
stretch
(page 101)

33 knee hug stretch
(page 96)

aDVaNCeD
FULL-BODY WORKOUT

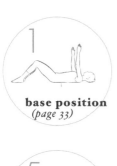
1

base position
(page 33)

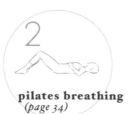
2

pilates breathing
(page 34)

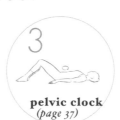
3

pelvic clock
(page 37)

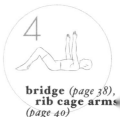
4

bridge *(page 38),*
rib cage arms
(page 40)

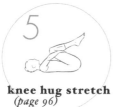
5

knee hug stretch
(page 96)

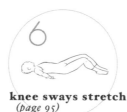
6

knee sways stretch
(page 95)

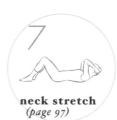
7

neck stretch
(page 97)

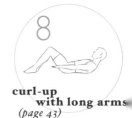
8

**curl-up
with long arms**
(page 43)

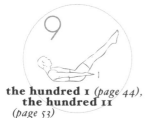
9

the hundred I *(page 44),*
the hundred II
(page 53)

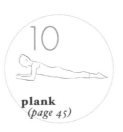
10

plank
(page 45)

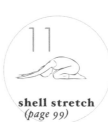
11

shell stretch
(page 99)

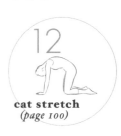
12

cat stretch
(page 100)

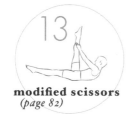
13

modified scissors
(page 82)

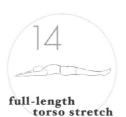
14

**full-length
torso stretch**
(page 98)

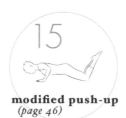
15

modified push-up
(page 46)

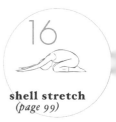
16

shell stretch
(page 99)

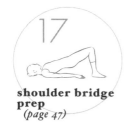
17

**shoulder bridge
prep**
(page 47)

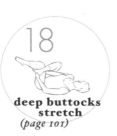
18

**deep buttocks
stretch**
(page 101)

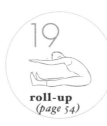
19

roll-up
(page 54)

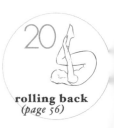
20

rolling back
(page 56)

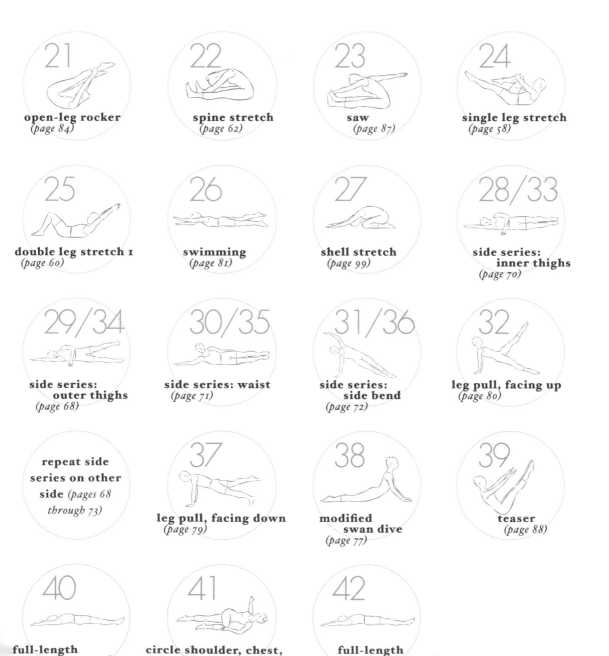

21
open-leg rocker
(page 84)

22
spine stretch
(page 62)

23
saw
(page 87)

24
single leg stretch
(page 58)

25
double leg stretch 1
(page 60)

26
swimming
(page 81)

27
shell stretch
(page 99)

28/33
side series:
inner thighs
(page 70)

29/34
side series:
outer thighs
(page 68)

30/35
side series: waist
(page 71)

31/36
side series:
side bend
(page 72)

32
leg pull, facing up
(page 80)

repeat side
series on other
side *(pages 68
through 73)*

37
leg pull, facing down
(page 79)

38
modified
swan dive
(page 77)

39
teaser
(page 88)

40
full-length
torso stretch
(page 98)

41
circle shoulder, chest,
and back stretch
(page 102)

42
full-length
torso stretch
(page 98)

ToTaL BoDY
RELAXATION STRETCH ROUTINE

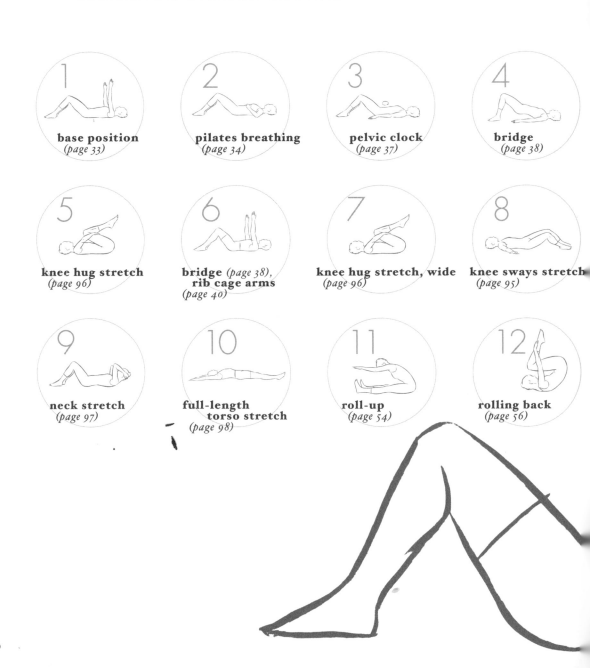

1 base position
(page 33)

2 pilates breathing
(page 34)

3 pelvic clock
(page 37)

4 bridge
(page 38)

5 knee hug stretch
(page 96)

6 bridge *(page 38)*,
rib cage arms
(page 40)

7 knee hug stretch, wide
(page 96)

8 knee sways stretch
(page 95)

9 neck stretch
(page 97)

10 full-length
torso stretch
(page 98)

11 roll-up
(page 54)

12 rolling back
(page 56)

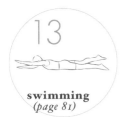

swimming
(page 81)

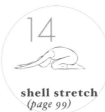

shell stretch
(page 99)

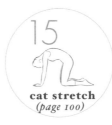

cat stretch
(page 100)

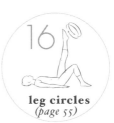

leg circles
(page 55)

knee hug stretch
(page 96)

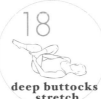

**deep buttocks
stretch**
(page 101)

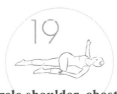

**circle shoulder, chest,
and back stretch**
(page 102)

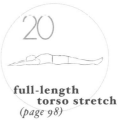

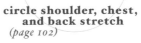

**full-length
torso stretch**
(page 98)

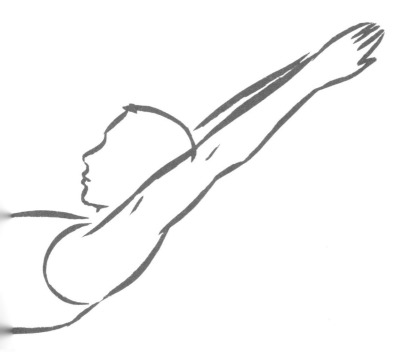

NiGHTTiMe
WIND-DOWN ROUTINE

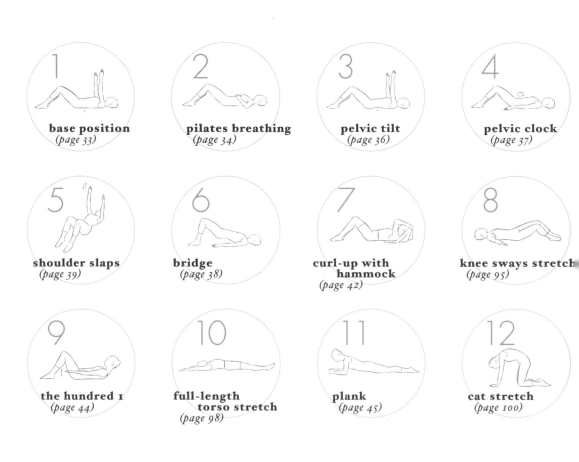

1 base position
(page 33)

2 pilates breathing
(page 34)

3 pelvic tilt
(page 36)

4 pelvic clock
(page 37)

5 shoulder slaps
(page 39)

6 bridge
(page 38)

7 curl-up with hammock
(page 42)

8 knee sways stretch
(page 95)

9 the hundred 1
(page 44)

10 full-length torso stretch
(page 98)

11 plank
(page 45)

12 cat stretch
(page 100)

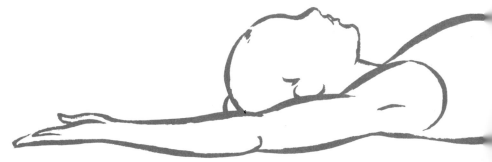

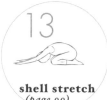

shell stretch
(page 99)

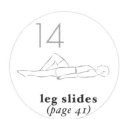

leg slides
(page 41)

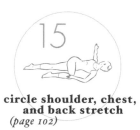

**circle shoulder, chest,
and back stretch**
(page 102)

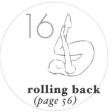

rolling back
(page 56)

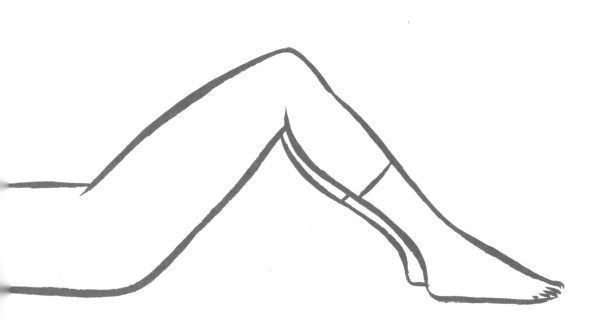

chapter 8

LiViNG PILATES FUSION:
BEYOND THE MAT

> Body and mind are not two and not one.
>
> {D.T. Suzuki}

Many people believe that they don't have time to take care of themselves. We all lead full, busy lives—juggling families, careers, personal relationships, and community activities. But because we are so busy, it's absolutely essential that we carve out time to care for ourselves. In the long run we'll be much better armed to pursue our passions and responsibilities. Think of it this way: you don't have time *not* to take care of yourself. When we neglect our bodies, we increase our risk of illness and other health problems. Taking care of ourselves today not only helps us enjoy the moment but also helps us enjoy life for many years to come.

There will be many times when you do not feel like practicing. It may seem like just another thing on your to-do list. That's when you need to take a look at what's going on in your life and ask yourself why you're feeling that way. Develop a habit of checking in with your inner feelings. Be alone for a moment and listen to what your body is saying to you. When you are feeling worn out, honor that feeling by doing gentle stretches and breathing for relaxation. If you are feeling anxious or full of nervous energy, take a brisk walk and engage in a more vigorous workout. Match your exercise routines to your moods. Respect your body's need to balance both work and rest.

Keep in mind that, as much as your body talks to you, it also listens very closely. Be mindful of what you say to your body. Treat it with kindness and respect. Your body absorbs all the messages it receives.

Try this quick test:

- Go into a stretch and reach the limit of your range of motion.
- Gently tell your muscles that they are safe and that you will only allow your muscles to go as far as they want.
- Asssure your body that your mind will not push but will instead follow.

You will likely find that once you have this little "body talk" you easily relax into a deeper stretch.

Scientists are only beginning to understand the intricacies of our vast mind-body communication network. Although we may not know all the scientific answers, we can find the answers within ourselves—if we choose to listen to our inner voice. Open your ears wide to hear this voice. Send positive messages, too. Align your positive thoughts with your values and goals. Channel all your power toward what you want. As you continue to train and build wellness of body, mind, and spirit, profound changes will occur.

The Pilates Fusion program lets you start exactly where you are now. It doesn't matter what shape you're currently in or how many minutes you work out—what matters is actually absorbing yourself in the practice a little bit every day. By learning how to focus your mind in the present, you begin to release the past and let go of self-blame. Remind yourself that each day brings you a fresh start.

Your daily choices are far more powerful than you may realize in creating optimal health. So keep it up! Through regular practice of Pilates Fusion you are choosing to affirm your life—each day is a wonderful gift. Treasure the value of life.

If you have been practicing Pilates Fusion for several weeks or months, you may now love your routines simply for that great post-workout feeling. In addition, be mindful of how your Pilates Fusion practice is enhancing your life. Are you feeling more energetic? Has your posture improved? Is your stomach flatter? Are you releasing more tension and relaxing more often? Do you feel more confident? Are you experiencing other benefits that you hadn't even considered before?

Keep in touch with what motivates you and what benefits you are receiving from your practice. When you can feel and see the rewards, you are much more likely to continue to make your practice an essential part of your life. Stay in tune with yourself and you will continue to meet with success.

index

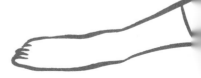

acknowledgments

A huge heartfelt thank you to the many people who helped to make this book possible. Thank you to my agent, Carol Roth, and to my editor, Jodi Davis, both for their enduring support to give this project life. Thank you to my mother and to my father for instilling in me since childhood an appreciation for the value of the richness of my cultural legacy that includes East Asian, American, and European influences. I especially appreciate all my many Pilates students and teachers who have led me to become a better teacher and supporter of all who seek to improve their well being. A big thank you to my brother, Ken Iwama, and to Kay McGuire for assisting with the photography for the exercise illustrations. Thanks always to Georgia, Anthony, and Mia, and to Marirose at m.rose sportswear for their constant support and faith in me.

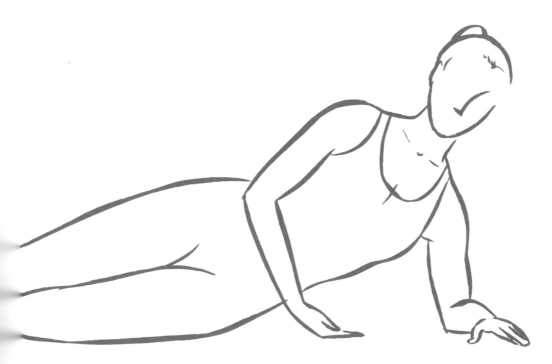

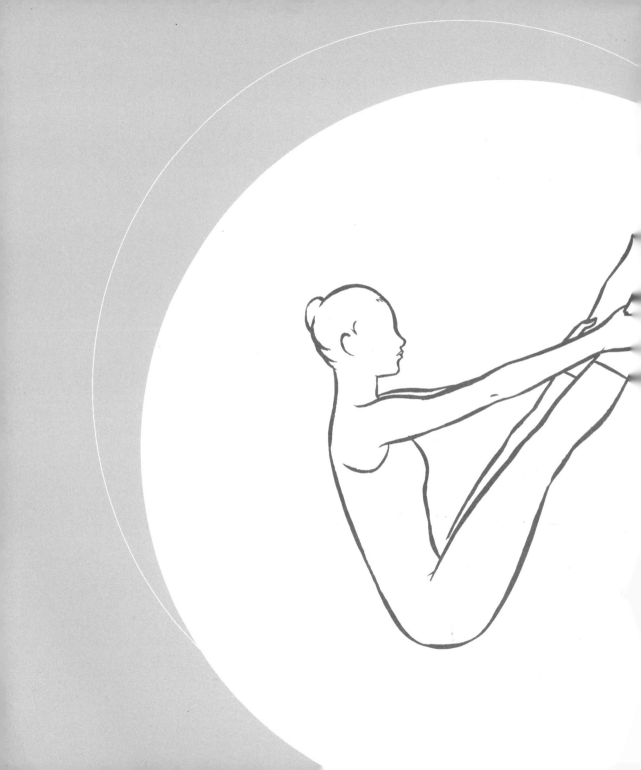